There are many superb bo
tions but there are few or
them, and none written ei
students or doctors. There
an expert surgical assistar
Normally, they can only be
way, by spending years in

This book describes the
systematic way, in surgery
different speciality areas. ,
for clinical-level medical st
other people who assist at s
including general practition
surgical technologists, will als
Whether planning a career in st
aiming for high marks in a surgic
are few better ways to impress a st
skilfully assisting at surgical operati

**Dr Comus Whalan** is a Visiting Surgeon,
Health Service, Adelaide, South Australi

# Assisting at Surgical Operations

## A Practical Guide

Edited by

### Comus Whalan BMBS MD FRACS

Visiting Surgeon, Noarlunga Health Service, Adelaide, South Australia

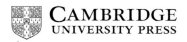
CAMBRIDGE
UNIVERSITY PRESS

CAMBRIDGE UNIVERSITY PRESS

Cambridge, New York, Melbourne, Madrid, Cape Town, Singapore, São Paulo

Cambridge University Press
The Edinburgh Building, Cambridge CB2 2RU, UK

Published in the United States of America by Cambridge University Press, New York

www.cambridge.org
Information on this title: www.cambridge.org/9780521680813

First published 2006
Typeset by Charon Tec Ltd, Chennai, India
www.charontec.com

Printed in the United Kingdom at the University Press, Cambridge

*A catalogue record for this publication is available from the British Library*

*Library of Congress Cataloguing in Publication data*

ISBN-13 978-0-521-68081-3 hardback
ISBN-10 0-521-68081-6 hardback

# Contents

# Contributors

**Amal Abou-Hamden** MBBS
Registrar, Department of Neurosurgery, Royal Adelaide Hospital,
North Terrace, Adelaide 5000, South Australia

**Elinor Atkinson** MBBS FRANZCOG
Senior Consultant Obstetrician and Gynaecologist, Flinders Medical Centre,
Flinders Drive, Bedford Park, Adelaide, South Australia

**Martin Bruening** BMBS MS FRCS(Ed) FRACS
Consultant Surgeon, The Queen Elizabeth Hospital,
Woodville Rd., Woodville, Adelaide, South Australia
Visiting Surgeon, Port Augusta, South Australia

**Richard Douglas** MD FRACS FRACP MRCP
Fellow, Department of Otolaryngology-Head and Neck Surgery,
The Queen Elizabeth Hospital, Woodville, SA 5011, Australia

**Graham Fraenkel** BMBS FRANZCO FRACS
Consultant Ophthalmologist, Cataract and Laser Surgicentre,
195 North Terrace, Adelaide 5000, South Australia

**Craig Jurisevic** MBBS MS FRACS
Consultant Cardiothoracic Surgeon, Cardiothoracic Unit, Royal Adelaide Hospital,
Adelaide 5000, South Australia

**Christopher Kirby** BMBS FRCS FRACS
Consultant Paediatric Surgeon, Women's and Children's Hospital,
72 King William Rd., North Adelaide, Adelaide 5006, South Australia

**Graham J Offer** BSc(Hons) MBChB FRCS(Eng) FRCS(Plast)
Consultant Plastic and Reconstructive Microsurgeon,
Leicester Royal Infirmary, Leicester, England and Clinical Teacher, Leicester and
Warwick Medical Schools

**Kath Phillips** RGON
Specialist Radiology nurse, Waikato District Hospital, Hamilton, New Zealand

**Phil Puckridge** MBBS FRACS
Consultant Vascular Surgeon, Waikato District Hospital, Hamilton, New Zealand

**Peter Riddell** FRACS (General Surgery) and FRACS (Plastic and Reconstructive surgery)
Consultant Plastic Surgeon, Flinders Medical Centre,
Bedford Park, Adelaide, South Australia
and Visiting Surgeon, various rural hospitals in South-East Asia

**Steve Santoreneos** MBBS FRACS
Consultant Neurosurgeon, Department of Neurosurgery, Royal Adelaide Hospital,
North Terrace, Adelaide 5000, South Australia

**Angelique Swart** BSc(Hons) BMBS Dip RANZCOG
Senior Registrar, Department of Obstetrics and Gynaecology,
Flinders Medical Centre, Flinders Drive, Bedford Park,
Adelaide 5000, South Australia

**John van Essen** BMBS FRACS
Consultant Orthopaedic Surgeon, Wakefield Orthopaedic Clinic,
270 Wakefield St., Adelaide 5000, South Australia.
Visiting Orthopaedic Surgeon, Royal Adelaide Hospital and
The Queen Elizabeth Hospital, Adelaide, South Australia

**Comus Whalan** BMBS MD FRACS
Visiting Surgeon, Noarlunga Health Service, Adelaide, South Australia,
Visiting Surgeon, Flinders Private Hospital, Bedford Park, Adelaide, South Australia

**Peter-John Wormald** MD FRACS FRCS FCS (SA)
Professor, Department of Otolaryngology-Head and Neck Surgery,
The Queen Elizabeth Hospital, Woodville, SA 5011, Australia

# Foreword

Despite continual turmoil in medical structures and hierarchies, the surgeon remains the principal individual responsible for the performance of an operation within the confines of the operating theatre. While the ultimate decisions for the procedure and the conduct of the operation remain largely in the hands of the surgeon, the successful performance of any surgery requires a well-trained and committed team. This team involves not only anaesthetists, nursing staff, orderlies, but also the surgical assistant. When a team of such committed individuals are brought together for the performance of surgery, simple or complex, the outcomes will be optimised when the environment in which all are working is skilful, focussed and competent. To this end the surgical assistant needs to be well trained and familiar with not only the instruments, tools and techniques of the operating room, but also their role in providing expert assistance to the surgeon. This book provides the basic guide for aspiring assistants so they can better understand the equipment they are using and the purpose of their assistance at surgical interventions.

All surgeons have had to progress through a period of time as a surgical assistant. Some surgeons are able to rapidly train their assistants to provide the support and skill they require to make the operation they are performing look surprisingly easy. Other surgeons have little idea how to best utilise the assistant that is made available to them. As a trainee surgeon, my knuckles were repeatedly bruised by a surgeon quick to point out my faults by the use of instruments being applied to the back of my hand as I held the retractor! Other surgeons created an atmosphere in the operating room that was unnecessarily stressful, while others behaved in a fashion that was rude, condescending and insulting to a professional colleague. These individuals, while scarred on my memory, have done little to encourage one to assist well, involve oneself in a learning experience and gain satisfaction from the conduct of a well-orchestrated surgical procedure.

Assisting at operations is not necessarily second nature to many surgeons and, indeed, some very competent surgeons make appalling assistants. It is true, however, that the very best surgeons often make extraordinarily good assistants. They understand the important tissue planes, how to hold instruments to best display the anatomy, and are able to provide helpful guidance for a trainee or an experienced surgeon.

The need to focus on the skills required of excellent surgical assistance is long overdue. This book provides such a guide and will be of immense value to all levels of surgical practitioners. Beginners will gain some insight into the range of activities required of an assistant and the experienced surgeon will be able to reflect on their own practice and consider which aspects could be improved or modified.

**Prof. Guy Maddern**
*RP Jepson Professor of Surgery*
*University of Adelaide*
*Adelaide*
*South Australia*

# Preface

Assisting at a surgical operation is an important task, and one that in my opinion, is sometimes under-appreciated. Without a skilful surgical assistant, all operations become more difficult. This added difficulty may not matter much in simple operations, but in complex ones, it matters a great deal. It may make the difference between a complex operation being merely challenging for the surgeon, and it being unsafe or almost impossible. Most surgeons would be reluctant to perform a complex operation without skilful assistance.

Surgery, and assisting at surgery, is a manual craft. In any manual craft, no expert can be created by simply reading textbooks on the subject. However, it is my hope that this book will hasten the process. I hope that it will help the reader to acquire more rapidly, information that previously has largely been obtainable only in a haphazard manner by spending years in the operating theatre.

The purpose of this book is to describe the general principles and techniques, which help to make a skilful surgical assistant in any specialty of surgery. However, some surgical subspecialties do require of the assistant, certain additional skills, which are described in the relevant chapters by my subspecialist colleagues.

It is not the book's intention to describe particular operations in detail. Indeed, specific operations are only mentioned where they are useful as examples, or where the assistant has a specific important role. To include here, a comprehensive description of all the various surgical operations in all the surgical specialties would obviously require a very large (and therefore very expensive) set of texts. Furthermore, it would also merely duplicate information that is already easily available elsewhere, in a number of superb textbooks of operative surgery. The reader is referred to some of these in the section 'Suggested further reading'.

There are places in the text where I am unflattering to my fellow surgeons. This is because I believe an accurate portrait is more useful than a flattering one. My intention is neither to omit blemishes, nor to paint them bigger than they truly are. Nor do I suggest that every surgeon has all the blemishes described in this book, any more than every patient suffers from all known diseases. If any of my colleagues is offended by my descriptions, I respectfully suggest that, while he or she may be free of all these flaws, most of the rest of us are not so lucky.

The subspecialty chapters were written by my friends and colleagues, whose names appear alongside each. While I may have added, subtracted or altered a few sentences here and there in each chapter, I cannot claim credit as a co-author for any of them. Some of the wording may be mine, but the wisdom is theirs.

I do not claim to have devised any of the techniques described in this book. Rather, other surgeons taught them to me during my years of surgical training. I have merely written them down and drawn pictures of them.

I would like to thank my parents Mrs Elizabeth Whalan, and the late Emeritus Prof. Douglas Whalan, AM LLM PhD, for their love, understanding and encouragement; all my friends and colleagues who contributed to this book; the staff at Cambridge University Press, especially Peter Silver and Emma Pearce; the operating theatre staff at Noarlunga Hospital for allowing me to photograph surgical instruments; all the surgeons who trained me, for putting up with my undoubted imperfections, and my wife Ange for the same reason, but on a larger scale.

# Introduction to the operating theatre

# Part 1

## A note on terminology

In the United States, the term 'operating room' or 'OR' is used, while in Australia and the United Kingdom, it is referred to as an 'operating theatre'. In the author's opinion, the word 'room' is probably more accurate. Unfortunately, however, if you use this term in Australia, listeners may think that your only operative experience has consisted of watching American television programmes.

Confusion sometimes arises over the correct way to address surgeons. That is, some surgeons use the title 'Mister' while others use 'Doctor'. Since all surgeons are doctors, it might seem logical that they should all be addressed as 'Doctor', and indeed, in the United States and Canada this is the rule. However, in the United Kingdom, the Republic of Ireland and some Commonwealth countries, the title 'Mister' is usual. This custom arose for a good reason: until the nineteenth century, most surgeons were not doctors at all. That is, in the present-day system, in order to train as a surgeon, one must first graduate from medical school. Previously, this was not required; an apprenticeship system existed. The title 'Mister' is simply a customary reminder of those earlier times (Loudon, 2000). (Although some surgeons might argue that surgeons calling themselves 'Mister' are more correct than other medical practitioners calling themselves 'Doctor'. This is because the word 'doctor' is Latin for 'teacher', and there are those who argue that the title should therefore properly be reserved for people holding a doctorate degree, i.e. a Ph.D. or similar qualification.)

To make matters more confusing, the broad geographical rules described above are subject to much regional and even local variation. That is, in some hospitals, only some surgeons will use the title 'Mister'. For example, in some hospitals, it is customary to address only consultant surgeons as 'Mister', while senior registrars (even if fully qualified) are called 'Doctor'. Even then, some consultant surgeons in Commonwealth countries prefer to be addressed as 'Doctor', for a variety of reasons of their own. Most female surgeons use the title 'Doctor', but some prefer 'Miss' or occasionally 'Mrs' or 'Ms'.

Although these may seem petty matters, some surgeons are offended by being addressed as 'Doctor', while others equally dislike being addressed as 'Mister'. The only reliable way to know the preferred form of address is to ask either the surgeon, or some other reliable local source.

This book refers throughout, to 'the assistant' at surgical operations. However, at some operations, more than one assistant may be present. Sometimes this is simply to teach more people, but at larger operations, it is often because more than one extra pair of hands is needed. In this case, the assistants are often given the specific titles of 'first assistant', 'second assistant' and so on. These roles imply certain positions at the operating table. Exactly where that position is, will vary depending on the operation, but the first assistant is the person who is most directly involved in assisting the main surgeon (e.g. by providing counter-traction, see p. 51). The second assistant usually has a less active role, for example holding retractors and cutting suture material, sometimes interspersed with periods of relative inactivity. It is best to establish beforehand, who is to be first or second assistant. This helps both assistants to avoid feeling an uncomfortable uncertainty about 'who should do what'.

A third reason for more than one assistant being present, is simply that the operation is done in two parts with two primary surgeons, each with their own assistant(s). In this case, each primary surgeon may have first, second and subsequent assistants. Each team may operate simultaneously (if operating in different parts of the body), or sequentially (if operating in the same area), or a combination of both. Examples of operations involving two primary surgeons operating simultaneously, include abdomino-perineal resections of the rectum (where the abdominal and perineal parts are performed simultaneously), and many oesophagectomies (where the thoracic and abdominal parts are performed simultaneously). An example of a sequential operation, is a major resection of a cancer of the oropharynx, where the cancer is resected by a team of ear, nose and throat surgeons, and the resultant defect is repaired by plastic-reconstructive surgeons.

# General conduct in the operating theatre

## ■ Relationship with theatre staff

Just like people anywhere else, theatre staff will usually react favourably to being treated like human beings instead of automatons. Like most normal people, if you are kind to them, they will help you. Often they teach you useful things about the operating theatre, which surgeons do not know. Just about everyone in an operating theatre is expert at something. Even the unassuming theatre orderlies usually know quite a lot about the various machines in the theatre. They are sometimes the only people who can fathom the mysteries of obscure operating table functions.

The words 'please' and 'thank you' are not commonly used during operations. This is not because surgeons have an abrupt, impolite manner (although unfortunately, some of them do), but rather because it eliminates words that may be mis-heard, and so makes a request easier to understand. That said, simple politeness seldom annoys people, so it is not wrong to say 'please' and 'thank you' if you speak clearly.

If you are on your first trip to the operating theatre, you may feel unsure about how to do some apparently simple things. In this case, the best thing to do is simply ask for advice from an experienced staff member. This particularly applies to scrubbing, gowning and gloving (see p. 36–42). You may be proud of the fact that you are already capable of washing your hands and dressing yourself unaided. However, these seemingly simple acts are done in the operating theatre in ways that vary subtly but importantly from the way they are done elsewhere. You will almost certainly do them wrongly the first time, if you do not ask someone to supervise you.

Always try to conduct yourself in a friendly, professional way. For example, be respectful to patients, even when they are under general anaesthetic. This is for at least three reasons. Firstly, and most importantly, it is simply professional courtesy. Secondly, if you have walked into the operating theatre after the operation has started, it is possible to believe mistakenly that a patient is under general anaesthetic, when he or she is under regional anaesthetic such as a spinal. Thirdly, it is possible that a patient under general anaesthetic will still be able to hear you and remember what you say. This poorly understood phenomenon, known as awareness, is thankfully rare, occurring in about one to two cases per thousand (Sebel *et al.*, 2004).

A careless unkind remark about the patient's physique under either of the second two circumstances may haunt you for a long time. A simple rule is to avoid saying anything in the presence of an anaesthetised patient, which you would not say if he or she were awake.

An extension of this point, is that it is best to avoid making comments suggesting that the operation is not proceeding well. In particular, comments suggesting that the surgeon is not doing a good job are almost never helpful. If the patient is awake, either one of these types of remarks will cause him or her great anxiety. Even if the patient is under deep general anaesthesia, such remarks will not endear you to the surgeon.

**Punctuality**  helps to create an illusion of excellence, even where none exists. Operating theatres are extremely expensive to run (perhaps £35 (US $70) per minute, depending on the method of calculation used), so if you are asked to assist at an operation, try to ensure you arrive on time. If you are early, make the most of your time. Familiarise yourself with the patient and the disease (see 'Preparing for operation' p. 21). It is important to realise that, once you have agreed to assist at an operation, this is a commitment that should not be broken. If you have other important engagements (such as tutorials), into which the operation may run, you must explain to the parties involved in this second commitment, that you may be delayed. It is inexcusable to desert a patient (and surgeon) and leave them without an assistant.

**Delays**  in starting an operation are very common in the operating theatre, and sometimes these can be for several hours. There are innumerable reasons for this. For example, an important pre-operative blood test may not yet be available, the patient may not have fasted for the required time, or the theatre may still be occupied by a previous operation that has taken longer than expected. Therefore, if you are studying, it is worth making up and carrying with you, pocket-sized cards with study topics summarised on them. Anatomy topics are particularly useful, because a lot of information can be put on one small card or diagram. That way, if you are delayed, and have run out of things to do, you can read these and so not waste time. Obviously, you can also use the cards anywhere else where you may have a few idle minutes (e.g. standing in a queue at the supermarket). Alternatively, you may use a hand-held computer for the same purpose.

The general way in which most operations are done, does not vary much between one surgeon and another, and even between one continent and another. However, surgeons sometimes attach a good deal of significance to these little variations. Indeed, some can become quite displeased at any variation from their routine, even if this variation may be perfectly reasonable practice. Although as an assistant, you may feel that the surgeon's displeasure is petty or even childish, it is best just to accept it. The reason it occurs is mostly that the surgeon has found a particular method works well in his or her hands. Therefore, he or she becomes reluctant to try a different method, which may not work so well. Your path will be smoother if you learn 'your' surgeon's routine.

## ■ Medio tutissimus ibis. [The middle course is safest and best.]

Ovid (b. 43 BC) [in Bulfinch, 1919]

This ancient quotation applies today in the operating theatre, as it does in many situations in life outside it. It is something of a recurring theme in this book. For example, it applies when cutting sutures (p. 57), when providing counter-traction (p. 51), when releasing clips (p. 82) and when 'following' sutures (p. 88). It also particularly applies to: (a) how active you should be as an assistant, (b) 'stress' and (c) talking in the operating theatre. These topics are discussed further below.

### Activity versus passivity

When assisting at operations, try to steer the middle course between being a passive retractor-holder, and being overly helpful to the point that you become intrusive and the surgeon feels you are trying to take over the operation. This is comparable to a good restaurant waiter, who steers the middle course between ignoring customers (on the one hand), and omnipresence (on the other). Sometimes this can be difficult, but generally, how closely you steer between passivity and activity depends on how experienced you are in comparison to the surgeon. Occasionally, when the assistant is very experienced (e.g. when a consultant is assisting a registrar), it can be difficult to tell who is the assistant and who is the primary operator. Early in your career, it is better to err on the side of being unobtrusive.

### Stress

For obvious reasons, an operating theatre can be a stressful place, not only to the patients entering it, but also to staff working there. Psychologists tell us that people perform tasks at their best when they are neither over-stressed, nor so under-stressed that they are bored. Therefore, try to keep yourself in the middle ground, even if others around you are not. This applies both to other staff members, including the surgeon, and to the patient. Remember that an operation that seems minor or even trivial to the staff, is not trivial to the patient (See also 'Concentrate on your task', p. 24).

## Talking in the operating theatre

Although this may seem a trivial topic, it is not. The impression you create amongst the operating theatre staff is probably as much dependent on what you say, and when you say it, as what you do. Continuous light-hearted banter during a difficult operation will annoy even the most placid surgeon. On the other hand, unwavering monastic silence may make you seem timid and unsociable.

It can be difficult to know when to talk and when not to. Generally, this will depend on a number of factors, some of which are obvious, but some of which are not. These factors include the surgeon's individual preference, the complexity of the operation about to be performed, and whether or not it is an emergency. For example, some surgeons insist on absolute silence while they are operating, while at the other end of the spectrum, some surgeons seem to prefer the continuous sound of music, or their own voice. Most occupy the middle ground, where talking is only unwelcome during some parts of the operation.

Even travelling to work prior to a complex operation such as a pancreatico-duodenectomy ('Whipple's procedure'), most surgeons will be thinking about the operation and will not be particularly interested in light social banter. Their mood is a little similar to students about to sit an examination. This seemingly unsociable attitude will also show itself during the 'tricky bits' which are usually found in the middle of any operation, but may be absent once that part is over (see 'general stages common to all operations' p. 30).

If you feel the need to speak during an operation, you may find it helpful to pause first, and classify your intended conversational subject matter into categories in order of importance. For example, your intended topic may be one of the following:

1 Important things you must say immediately, if you think a serious mistake is about to be made, for example 'an instrument may be left in the abdomen if we close it now'.
2 Questions you would like to ask about the operation.
3 General information about the patient, or about medicine in general.
4 Unrelated social banter.

Having classified your intended topic, decide if it is appropriate to the setting.

It is perfectly reasonable to ask a surgeon prior to an operation, whether or not you can ask questions during it.

## ■ Pagers and mobile (cell) phones

These devices inevitably cause disturbance, and some surgeons even ban them from the operating theatre while they are operating. Unless it is essential that you be contactable immediately (e.g. if you are on emergency call), try to keep them either outside the operating theatre, diverted elsewhere, or switched off.

In some operating theatres, clerical staff at the front desk are employed to answer pagers and mobile phones belonging to staff in the operating theatre. Otherwise, if you are at the operating table, other nursing or medical staff in the theatre must answer them for you. This can sometimes create friction: the other staff may sometimes resent answering your calls, because it interrupts their other proper duties, and because they feel (with some justification) that they are being used as your personal secretary. Therefore, if you find yourself with no alternative but to take your pager or mobile phone into the operating theatre, other staff will be much more understanding if you explain your situation, and apologise in advance for any inconvenience it may cause.

For some reason, the location of a ringing pager or mobile phone can be surprisingly difficult to pinpoint by ear. Consequently, if there is more than one pager or mobile phone in the theatre, staff may have difficulty working out which one is ringing. Therefore, the devices are best kept a metre or two apart, but so that they are easily visible. Although this may seem a small point, when you are dependent on someone else doing you a favour to answer your pager, it saves him or her the irritation of having to pick up several different pagers, simply to discover which one is ringing.

Surgeons often forget to remove mobile phones and pagers from their pockets before scrubbing. This means that when the device rings, other staff in the operating theatre must rummage around in the surgeon's pockets in the middle of an operation. This is usually slightly embarrassing to both rummager and rummagee. If you are so fond of your device that you must have it in your pocket, the back pocket of your scrubs is probably the easiest place from which to retrieve it.

## ■ Food and drink

These are not permitted in the operating theatre, although of course they are encouraged in the tea-room. It is wise to enter the operating theatre with a full stomach and an empty bladder whenever possible. This is especially so when the case you are about to assist at may take several hours. Although this may seem obvious, one is often in a rush to 'get to theatre'. It is too easy to omit a sandwich and quick glass of sustaining beverage, and so condemn yourself to spending the next few hours feeling uncomfortable. As a consequence, your enjoyment of and learning from the operation will be decreased, as will your ability to concentrate on the task. Except in dire emergencies, few will begrudge you a quick break.

## ■ If you feel faint

It is common for this to occur early on in your career. Presumably, it occurs from the hypotensive effects of standing still for long periods in a warm environment, coupled with the mediaeval spectacle of human viscera on open display. While faintness is embarrassing, it is far better to admit to it early on, and be excused to sit down, rather than try to continue and then fall face-first into the surgical wound.

The risk of faintness can be reduced, though not eliminated, by ensuring you are well hydrated before entering the operating theatre. Periodically contracting your leg muscles may also help, by reducing venous pooling. Because of the obvious need to wear standardised theatre clothes, little can be done to avoid overheating by modifying your clothing. You may improve matters slightly by wearing cooler underwear (especially, avoiding thermal underwear), and perhaps by choosing a cloth gown rather than a waterproof one.

## ■ Know dimensions

During an operation, it is common for a surgeon to ask that you place an instrument in a certain site, with an accompanying description in centimetres or millimetres. In particular, surgeons often request that a suture be cut to a certain specified length (e.g. half a centimetre). Although it is only a small point, when you have a spare moment outside the operating theatre, it is useful to check with a ruler, that you know how long half a centimetre is. This seems to be one of those odd facts, which we often think we know, when we do not. That way, when you are asked to cut a suture a certain length, you will be able to do so reasonably accurately. A rough guide, which can be used intra-operatively, is that an average adult man's index finger is about 2 cm broad at the distal phalanx.

# Universal Precautions

It hardly needs stating that it is possible to acquire disease from your patient during an operation. 'Universal Precautions' is the name given to a set of recommendations which are aimed at minimising the risk of this occurring in the operating theatre and elsewhere. The recommendations mainly aim to reduce transmission of blood-borne viral diseases such as HIV/AIDS and the various forms of hepatitis, especially Hepatitis B and C. However, there are other diseases (both known and as yet unknown) against which Universal Precautions will, or at least should, help to protect you. The key principle of Universal Precautions is that every person should be treated as though he or she has one of these diseases, regardless of his or her known or supposed infection status. In the operating theatre, Universal Precautions measures include double-gloving, and wearing a waterproof gown, a mask and proper eye protection such as an eye shield or safety glasses.

## ■ Transmissible disease in the operating theatre

This can occur in several different ways, but the commonest are needle-stick injuries and splash of body fluids into the eye. Infection can also be transmitted by the patient's body fluids coming into contact with an open wound (e.g. a cut on the finger with a hole in the glove). For this reason, it is strongly recommended that you follow your hospital's policy on immunisation. Most hospitals advise that you should be immunised against Hepatitis B.

## ■ If you suffer a needle-stick injury

Most hospitals have an Occupational Health and Safety Department, and in the larger ones, there is usually a member of that department available after normal office hours. Most hospitals also have standard protocols to be followed in the event of a needle-stick injury. It is strongly recommended that you follow your hospital's protocol. However, most recommend you should immediately encourage bleeding from the site, for example by squeezing it, and then wash the area thoroughly with soap and warm water. Do not use a scrubbing brush.

After these basic first-aid measures, record the patient's name and hospital record number, and report the event promptly to your Occupational Health and Safety Department. In most hospitals, a blood sample for serology will be taken from you, and from the patient involved, with a follow-up appointment some months later.

## ■ If you suffer an eye splash

Irrigate the eye and surrounding area with tap water. After these immediate first-aid measures, the procedure is broadly similar to that for needle-stick injury.

# Clothing in the operating theatre

Operating theatres are designed to ensure the operation site can be kept sterile (or perhaps more accurately, to minimise contamination from the external environment). Several features help with this. For example, the theatres are kept extremely clean, with frequent dusting and mopping. In most, the corners of the room are rounded to enable them to be cleaned easily. The air is filtered to remove bacteria-carrying particles, and flows in specific directions from the operating theatre outwards.

## ■ Scrubs

Special clothes, often known as 'scrubs' or 'blues', are worn in the operating theatre. Their main purpose is to decrease the transmission of micro-organisms, both from the staff to the patient, and vice-versa. Scrubs are provided by the hospital, and are usually found on racks either just inside or just outside the operating theatre's change-rooms. Like normal clothes, you simply wear your underwear beneath them. To prevent your normal street clothes from carrying dust and micro-organisms into the operating theatres, you must change into scrubs before entering. In most operating theatre suites, there is a line clearly marked on the floor, beyond which you may not pass unless wearing scrubs, and the correct hat and footwear.

Scrubs are usually blue or green in colour, because these colours are restful to the eye. Generally, the choice lies between overalls, or trousers and a shirt. Female change-rooms may also stock skirts and dresses. A wide range of sizes is usually provided. The size is usually marked on each garment, often on the 'badge area' of the chest. When you have worked out which size fits you best, try to remember it for next time. However, there is often only a loose correlation between the stated size of a scrub garment, and its actual size. Therefore, once you have found a garment that you suspect will fit you, it is wise to check this by simply holding the garment against your body, before putting it on.

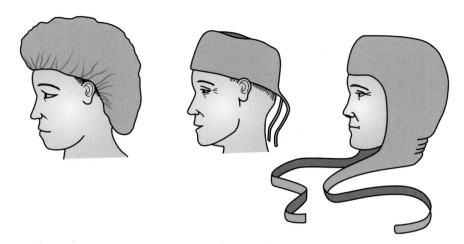

**Figure 3.1** Different styles of surgical hat. From left to right: the elasticated cap, the plain cap and the balaclava.

You may find that none of the sizes fits you very well. In this case, choose a size that is too loose rather than too tight, because you will be more comfortable. You may feel that you look slightly silly, but it is unlikely that anyone else will notice because surgical scrubs are not high-fashion items, and because half the other people in the operating theatre will be doing the same thing themselves.

Scrubs do not need to be changed after each operation, unless they are particularly soiled. Instead, they are discarded for cleaning at the end of each operating list.

## ■ Other operating theatre clothing

### Hat

There are several different types, such as the plain cap, the elasticated cap and the balaclava style (see Figure 3.1). The tapes of the plain cap are simply tied over the occipital area, while those of the balaclava are crossed around the neck first. The elasticated cap is held in place by an elastic rim.

There seems to be no agreement as to which hat is best, and in most operating theatres, the type you choose is largely a matter of individual preference. However, some surgeons prefer one type over others, to the point that they insist all staff entering their operating theatre wear that type of hat. For example, in orthopaedic surgery (and especially major joint replacement surgery), surgeons usually prefer the balaclava type.

The elasticated cap can be worn comfortably with the elastic either above or below the ears. If you wear this type of hat, do not wear it with the elastic sitting

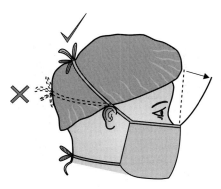

**Figure 3.2** How to tie the face mask. Note that the upper tie is tied high above the occiput and the transparent plastic splashguard is flipped away from the face to minimise fogging.

*on* the ears, because it can become quite uncomfortable, and you will be unable to adjust it once scrubbed. If you have long hair, you should wear the elasticated cap or the balaclava, and avoid the plain cap, because it will not keep your hair in place well.

## Face mask

Whether or not a surgical mask makes any difference to wound infection rates is unclear (Lipp and Edwards 2002). However, there is good evidence that it decreases the number of bacteria in the air in the operating theatre, and indisputably it will help protect you from body fluid splashes to your face, so you should wear one. There are several different designs. The author prefers the sort with a clear plastic splashguard. Some people find that the splashguard tends to fog up with condensation from the wearer's breath, but if you pinch the upper wire across your nose, and flip the visor a little away from your face, this does not usually occur (see Figure 3.2).

Most masks are secured in place by two pairs of tapes: an upper and lower pair. The lower pair should simply be tied at the back of your neck. The upper pair should be tied over your hat.

The natural tendency is to tie the upper pair over your neck, but for some reason, they seem to sit better if they are tied over the occipital area. Mould the mask gently around your jaw.

## Eye protection

Sometimes this is included in the mask (the plastic splashguard described above). Alternatively, you may wear safety glasses. Most operating theatres provide these on a loan basis.

If you wear glasses, you may find that your breath causes them to fog up in the operating theatre. To avoid this problem, use a plain mask (i.e. the type of mask that has no plastic splashguard). Then apply a piece of wound-dressing tape (e.g. 'Micropore' or 'Transpore') about 15 cm in length horizontally along the upper border of the mask, so that the tape sticks the mask to your facial skin. This prevents the breath from venting upwards onto the glasses.

While this method is usually highly effective, unfortunately the tape is often painful to remove afterwards. However, this latter problem can be eased by making the tape less sticky before using it. Do this by simply applying it to your clothing and peeling it off again several times, before applying it to your face.

## Footwear

Regular visitors to the operating theatre usually have their own footwear, which is kept in the change-room. The variety is large, but surgeons most commonly wear rubber boots or clogs. However, almost all theatres also provide overshoes of paper or cloth. These are simply slipped over your normal shoes. It is best to avoid wearing someone else's boots or clogs. Apart from the hygiene issues, their owner will not thank you for wearing them.

Like scrubs themselves, overshoes are discarded after each theatre session, or sooner if they become soiled. If you do have your own theatre boots and they become soiled, some operating theatres will clean them for you if you leave them in a particular place (usually a trolley in the change-room). In other theatres, you must clean them yourself.

## Jewellery

Operating theatres usually require that you remove most, if not all jewellery. This particularly applies to ear-rings, which could potentially fall into the wound, and watches and rings, which probably make surgical scrubbing less effective. However, there is some evidence to suggest that removing pierced ear-rings and nose-rings increases local bacterial counts. It may be preferable to cover these items with hat and mask instead of removing them.

To lessen the chance of losing a ring, simply put it in your wallet. Alternatively, if you have a buckle-style watchstrap, thread the ring on the watchstrap and put it in your pocket. If not, tape the ring to your watchstrap.

Nail polish is discouraged in the operating theatre, on the grounds that microscopic imperfections in the nail polish may harbour micro-organisms. Nevertheless, the little scientific evidence that exists, does not support this theory (Arrowsmith *et al.*, 2001).

Long fingernails are somewhat impractical for surgical assisting because they impair manual dexterity and because they can hole theatre gloves. If in doubt, ask the policy in your operating theatre.

## ■ Re-entering the operating suite

Different hospitals have different policies on what is required when leaving and re-entering the theatre suite for short periods of time (e.g. a brief visit to the cafeteria or ward). However, at the very least, most will ask that when leaving, you remove your theatre shoes, and don an over-garment, such as a white coat or patient gown. This is to decrease possible contamination of your scrubs by the world outside the operating theatre. Other hospitals are stricter, and in some, wearing scrubs outside the operating theatre is completely forbidden.

Clothes that look tidy and professional on the ward are mostly slower to change in and out of, than track-suit pants and a tee-shirt. Therefore, the desire to look professional on the ward may seem to act in opposition to the desire to arrive punctually in the operating theatre. However, there are number of simple tricks to help you overcome this. For example, if you do not have your own theatre boots, wear footwear that is quick to put on and off, such as slip-on boots rather than lace-ups. Even better, avoid the need to change footwear at all by wearing shoes that can slide completely through your trouser-legs without snagging. The point of snagging is usually at the heel. When leaving the operating theatre, this problem can be partly overcome by not removing theatre overshoes until after your street trousers are back on; the overshoes help the heel to slide through. Obviously, this should only be done with overshoes that are not soiled.

If you wear a shirt and tie, with a little practice you will find you can simply loosen the tie slightly, plus three or four buttons of the shirt, to enable you to slip the shirt and tie off and on again together, like a pullover rugby jersey. This avoids the need to re-knot the tie and button up the whole shirt.

While all the above manoeuvres will help you to save time, they are obviously a poor substitute for simply arriving five minutes earlier.

# 4 Personnel: who's who in the operating theatre

Because all staff in the operating theatre wear similar clothing (see Chapter 3), it can be difficult to know exactly who each person is. However, the staff can be divided into the following categories.

## ■ Doctors

These consist mostly of surgeons and anaesthetists. According to their level of seniority, each of these will be consultants, registrars, residents or interns. Depending on the complexity of the operation, the most senior surgeon may either perform the operation, or assist, or simply observe. Occasionally, other doctors may also be present. For example, a paediatrician is normally present at caesarean sections, ready to look after the baby. In some hospitals, a specially trained paediatric nurse is sometimes present instead.

## ■ Nurses

Nurses are allocated specific tasks for each operation, although often they are quite capable of doing more than one of these tasks. They include the following categories.

### Instrument nurses or 'scrub nurses'

The scrub nurse's main role is to keep the surgical instruments clean and ready for use, and pass them to the surgeon promptly when needed. Scrub nurses are especially trained to pass instruments into the surgeon's (or assistant's) hand in the correct orientation so that the instrument is ready for immediate use. This is very helpful, as it means you can simply ask for an instrument, extend your hand without taking your eye off the operation, and the instrument will be placed there.

Scrub nurses usually know the instruments extremely well, and are understandably protective of them. Consequently, they will not like it if you hoard instruments next to yourself, beyond their reach, just in case you need them later in the operation. Hoarding instruments is bad practice (see also p. 54–55).

When you return instruments to the scrub nurse, return them handle first. This is not only basic good manners, but is safer. Avoid the temptation to help yourself to instruments from the scrub nurse's trolley. This practice makes it much more difficult for the scrub nurse to keep track of the instruments, and most scrub nurses justifiably consider it an insult. Instead, ask for the instruments you want. You are being treated to table service, so do not turn it into a buffet.

### Scout nurses (known as 'runners' in the United Kingdom)

They are not scrubbed. They wait in the operating theatre to assist the scrub nurse, for example by fetching extra instruments or materials from storage areas. Often the scout and scrub nurses will alternate duties between cases.

### Anaesthetic nurses

As their name implies, they assist the anaesthetist. Their training and skills are different to the scout and scrub nurses, so they usually will not scrub.

## ■ Other personnel

### Theatre orderlies

Theatre orderlies help to move the patient around the operating theatre suite, and transfer them to and from the operating table. They are often expert at fixing problems with equipment, such as operating tables, diathermy machines and laparoscopic equipment.

### Radiographers

Radiographers operate X-ray and other equipment, such as Image Intensifiers and Ultrasound machines.

# The operation itself

# Part II

# Preparing for the operation

Whenever possible, try to read up in advance about the operation you will be assisting at (see also 'Key points', p. 34). Familiarise yourself with the patient. Try to ensure you understand the key points about the patient, the pathology and the proposed operation. What is the disease? Where is it? What symptoms has the patient had? What examination findings? What complications? What investigations? What other medical problems are there? In particular, are there any medical problems that may have an important effect on the surgery? For example, is the patient on warfarin? In an ideal world, you would read the case-notes as well as taking a thorough history and examining the patient yourself. Unfortunately, we live in a world that is often far from ideal, so you will often not have time to do this fully. Under these circumstances, it is probably better to spend more time with the patient, and only use the case-notes to clarify any points that your history and examination do not reveal.

If the pathology may be difficult to identify once the patient is anaesthetised, ensure it is clear beforehand, and the consent form is correct. This particularly applies to 'sided' operations (e.g. inguinal hernias, joint replacements), but also to some others where the pathology can disappear from view when the patient lies down (e.g. midline incisional hernias, varicose veins). It is often very helpful simply to ask the patient where he or she expects the operation site to be. Marking the site of the pathology with a skin-marking pen is also a wise safeguard in the above circumstances. This mark is often simply an arrow drawn pointing to the correct surgical site.

Some assistants initially find the idea of drawing such a mark on a patient, vaguely demeaning to the patient, perhaps thinking it to be reminiscent of marking an animal at an abattoir. However, once the reason for the mark is explained to them, most patients are pleased and reassured by it. Furthermore, in the author's opinion, having an ink arrow on the skin for a few hours is considerably less insulting to a patient, than operating on the wrong side.

It is helpful to know about the patient's social circumstances. It is good medical practice to know, for example, that the patient is a delivery-van driver, whose job sometimes entails lifting heavy crates, and who lives alone. Furthermore, knowing such details can also help you remember the patient on the ward. Rehearse those details to yourself during the operation. For example, think to yourself, 'We are operating on Mr Davis' hernia. He's a delivery-van driver who sometimes needs to lift heavy crates, and lives alone, so he may be unable to work for a few weeks post-operatively.' That way, when you review him the next day, he will not just be 'the bloke with the hernia we did yesterday', or worse, 'Er… who is he again?' He will be a real person.

Know the results of relevant investigations. Which tests are relevant will obviously depend on the patient and the operation. Broadly, you might classify the relevant investigations into those that describe the pathology itself, any potential complications of the pathology, and other investigations relevant to the general health of the patient. For example, for a patient being operated on for colon cancer, the investigations the surgeon will be particularly interested in will be:

*Pathology itself:* How was the diagnosis made? If it was by colonoscopy, read the colonoscopy report. Who did the colonoscopy? Where exactly is the cancer? That is, does the report give a reliable indication of the anatomical site of the cancer? Did the scope pass right to the caecum? (If not, the rest of the colon proximal to the cancer could contain other pathology, such as a second cancer, and will need to be assessed carefully intra-operatively). Has a biopsy confirmed cancer? If no colonoscopy has been done, what investigation diagnosed the cancer? Was it a sigmoidoscopy? A barium enema? A CT scan?

*Potential complications*: Are there any obstructive symptoms? Is the patient anaemic clinically, or on the blood picture? Is he or she malnourished? Is there a suggestion of extracolonic spread, such as abnormal liver enzymes, or imaging such as CT, liver ultrasound, or chest X-ray?

There is almost always an X-ray viewing box in the operating theatre; put relevant X-rays up on it. If there is a selection of imaging (and most X-ray packets contain far more sheets than can fit on a small viewing box), pick the most recent pictures that show the pathology. For example, if the patient is about to have a cholecystectomy, look for the ultrasound sheets showing gallbladder stones and the bile duct. Leave the sheets showing nice pictures of a normal spleen, kidneys and aorta. Occasionally, the radiologist reporting the films will have circled the pathology with a wax pencil (the 'radiological crayon sign'); this makes your task easier.

During the induction phase of anaesthesia (i.e. when the patient is 'going to sleep'), stay away from the patient, and avoid noise. Stimuli such as noise are disruptive to the smooth induction of anaesthetic, and will not endear you to the anaesthetist.

Check the shave (see p. 45). Is the correct area shaved? On the correct side, and with an adequate surrounding margin? Has the shaved hair been satisfactorily removed, or are tufts of it sitting on the skin, waiting to fall into an incision and cause a wound infection?

Insert a urinary catheter for long operations, and operations where fluid-balance monitoring is important during or after surgery.

Help position the patient, and put on thrombo-embolic compression devices, stockings or both.

Ensure the diathermy plate is in place safely (see also p. 76). It should make good contact with the skin, and be placed as close as reasonably practical to the operative site itself. It should also be placed away from bony prominences, and away from areas with poor blood supply, such as scar tissue. Typically, it is placed on the patient's thigh or less commonly, the abdomen. Occasionally, very hairy patients need to be shaved to allow the diathermy plate to stick properly.

# 6 General intra-operative principles

For all its complexities and apparent mystique, surgery is a manual craft. Therefore, the simple rules of any manual craft apply. For example, avoid doing anything that might distract the surgeon. Do not allow instruments or any part of your body, to obscure the surgeon's view of the operation. Keep unnecessary movements of your hands and vocal cords to a minimum. In particular, do not play with the instruments. Some assistants have even been known to dance to music playing on the radio; few surgeons will fail to be annoyed by this.

## ■ Concentrate on your task

Although surgical operations require the surgeon and assistant to concentrate continuously, the intensity of this varies. For example, while it is common for the surgeon and other staff members (including yourself) to chat about unrelated matters during straightforward parts of the operation, do not allow yourself to become distracted even at these times. This situation may be likened to driving a car; although it is reasonable to carry on a conversation while driving on an easy stretch of road, it is inadvisable to take your hands off the steering wheel and stop watching the road while doing so. Similarly, most operations have 'tricky bits' at some point (see p. 33). This is perhaps analogous to driving a car on a slippery road on a dark foggy night; both situations require full concentration.

If you are ever assisting a surgeon who is dealing with a massive bleed, or some other difficult problem, you must strive to remain calm and put all distractions from your mind. If you are inexperienced, it may be prudent to ask the surgeon tactfully, if he or she would like a more experienced assistant than yourself, if one is available. If the experienced assistant arrives, do not assume that is your cue to leave. On the contrary, your help as a second assistant will probably be highly valued. Even if your role may seem modest (like simply standing holding a retractor), every small help is useful when an operation is difficult. Therefore, stay at your position at least until the 'cavalry' has arrived, scrubbed, at the operating table, and do not leave without asking first.

## ■ Anticipation

This word is commonly used to describe the actions of a good surgical assistant. It is really another way of saying 'be prepared'. It means that you anticipate what the surgeon is going to do next, and are already prepared for this when it occurs, so that no time is wasted. Surgeons are usually busy people. Consequently, they almost universally seem to resent having even a few seconds of their time wasted unnecessarily. This trait manifests itself to a varying extent outside the operating theatre, but is at its most florid within it.

In some ways, anticipation starts before the operation. For example, if you have read about the operation beforehand in an operative text, and learnt its different steps, you will find it easier to predict what the surgeon is about to do next, and prepare for it.

Other examples of anticipation include:

- During the course of almost all operations, the site of the surgical action will move. For example, during the process of gaining access to a deeply placed surgical site (e.g. the aorta), the action becomes deeper, as more and more overlying tissue layers of skin, fat, fascia and muscle are divided or retracted. Once the organ of interest has been reached, the site of action will often continue to move. For example, during mobilisation of the right colon for a right hemicolectomy, the site of action will follow a line along the lateral border of the colon. During an umbilical hernia repair, the surgeon will usually dissect completely around the hernia sac, mobilising it from the surrounding fat. In this case, the site of surgical action describes a complete circle as it slowly circumnavigates the hernia sac.

  As an assistant, do not feel that you and your retractors must always remain frozen, statue-like, in one position until directed otherwise. While it is sometimes necessary, or even essential, to remain immobile when the site of surgical action is stationary, it is of no benefit to continue doing so when the site of the action has moved elsewhere. Instead, re-adjust your retractors so that you are providing the best view for the surgeon.

- When the surgeon is tying a suture, be ready to cut the suture when it is held up for you to do so. Do not wait for the surgeon to hold the suture up, and then ask the scrub nurse for the suture scissors. Instead, while the knot is being tied, obtain the scissors, and rest your hands in the cutting position (see Figure 6.1). If possible, hold the scissors with their tips about 10 cm away from the suture.

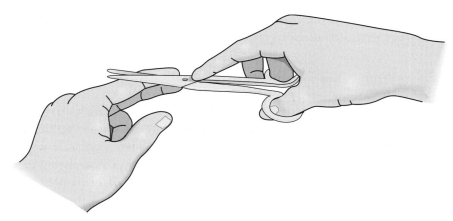

**Figure 6.1** Cutting sutures: hand position. The tips of the scissors are rested on the fingers of the left hand, to stabilise them.

As soon as the suture is held up for cutting, glide your hands quickly but smoothly forward and cut. But be certain the surgeon wants it cut and not clipped! (see p. 61).

- If the surgeon and yourself will be performing a 'clip and cut' manoeuvre, (see below and also p. 61), hold the clip in one hand, and the scissors in the other. This wastes less time than first applying the clip, and then reaching around for the scissors. Furthermore, if you can see that you will need several clips, you can ask the scrub nurse if you may have them all together. (This is one of the rare exceptions to the general rule against hoarding surgical instruments (see p. 17 and p. 54). If the scrub nurse passes them to you all together, it prevents the inconvenience of having to hand them to you one at a time. Moreover, because they will only be hoarded for a short time, it is unlikely they will be damaged.) You may find it convenient to clip the artery clips to the drapes in an unobtrusive spot, to secure them.

- During some operations, one surgical manoeuvre is repeated a number of times. When this occurs, it becomes easier to anticipate what the surgeon will do next. For example, when resecting part of the colon, the mesentery (the fatty skirt of the bowel attaching it to the back wall of the abdominal cavity) is repeatedly clipped and ligated. The usual method involves clipping the mesentery twice, then cutting between the clips: clip, clip, cut. Clip, clip, cut.

- Tactfully ask the scrub nurse for materials or instruments you will need, before you actually need them. For example, if the operation is ending, and the stage of closing the wound is approaching, it may be appropriate to ask the surgeon whether irrigation or a drain will be needed, and which suture material he or she would like to use to close the wound. Ask the scrub nurse if these materials are already on his or her trolley.

It is important to do this diplomatically, because most scrub nurses rightfully pride themselves on having such materials at the ready. This is particularly so when the scrub nurse has worked with an individual surgeon for some time, and the operation is a common or routine one. Under such circumstances, scrub nurses often know individual surgeon's preferences in considerable detail. Furthermore, most operating theatres have a 'preference card' system, whereby each individual surgeon's preferred instruments and suture material for each common operation, are written on a card. This allows the theatre staff to prepare the materials in advance.

## ■ Sharps

For safety reasons, sharp instruments ('sharps'), such as needles and scalpels, are not passed directly hand-to-hand, but via a special dish. Unsurprisingly, this is called the sharps dish. It is usually bright yellow, so it is easy to spot amongst all the other equipment. If you absolutely must pass a sharp instrument hand-to-hand, pass it handle first. Indeed, it is good manners to pass all instruments handle first. Do not pass instruments behind someone else's back, if you can avoid it. The person may not notice you doing it, and move backwards unexpectedly, causing contamination, or if a sharp instrument is being passed, possibly injury.

Do not be tempted to use your fingers as retractors in the wound; this will make the surgeon concerned about cutting you. Even if no sharp instrument is in use, an instrument is usually better than the fingers. An exception to this rule occurs when the surgeon is opening the abdomen with a midline incision (see p. 52–3).

## ■ Adjusting the light source

Unless it is obvious that the light is not directed properly at the operating field, ask the surgeon if he or she would like you to adjust it before actually doing so. Adjustment can be done in one of three ways:
1  Simply grasp the (sterile) handle, and aim the main operating light more directly into the area where the surgeon is operating.
2  Adjust the focus of the operating light. This enlarges or diminishes the size of the area that is lighted. In some models of operating light, you can do this by twisting the (sterile) light handle, while others must be adjusted by an unsterile third person, such as an orderly.

3. Recruit another light source. This may be a second mobile overhead light ('satellite'), or a light mounted on a headband on the surgeon's forehead. Rarely, a light on a stand may be needed.

## ■ Steady hands

Much is made of a surgeon's steady hands. However, there is far more to surgery than simply owning a pair of these. Contrary to what Hollywood scriptwriters may think, to do most operations properly, probably requires no more than average manual dexterity. In the author's opinion, anyone who can write neatly probably has enough manual dexterity to do most surgical operations. The qualities that distinguish a superior surgeon from an average one are far more subtle, reside in the cerebral cortex rather than the cerebellum, and mainly involve complex decision-making and judgement.

Nevertheless, you cannot do an operation properly, or assist effectively, if you are a clumsy oaf. To help you maximise your manual dexterity, several tips are given below.

Stand with your feet about shoulder-width apart. This will steady you. If possible, rest your pelvis or lower abdomen gently against the operating table. In effect, this forms a tripod with your two legs, stabilising the lower body (*cf.* scissor-grip, p. 56). Avoid bumping the table and leaning on the patient excessively.

Ergonomically, it is most comfortable to have your elbows flexed at about 90° when operating or assisting, and to have a straight, relaxed back. The operating table is normally adjusted to a height that suits the surgeon, which will not necessarily suit you, the assistant. If you are short, and the operating table is too high for you, ask for a step to stand on. These are portable stands of metal or plastic, typically about 10–15 cm high, designed specifically for this purpose. If you are tall and the table is low for you, your options are limited. Standing with your legs further apart helps a little, but you may simply have to accept a posture that is less than perfect.

Any delicate manual task is much harder if you hold your hand at arm's length, than if the arm is supported. Therefore, whenever possible, steady your hand (e.g. at the wrist level) on something else (see Figure 6.1).

Try to use both hands when assisting, rather than keeping one hand idle. Even if you are only holding one instrument, you will usually find that using both hands is less tiring, and allows you to steady the instrument more accurately.

Whenever possible, do not allow your hands to cross over each other.

Try to see what the surgeon is doing at all times, but without interfering with his or her view. Sometimes this is not possible when the surgeon is operating at the end of a deep narrow wound.

# ■ Improving the surgeon's view

In an open wound, try to give the surgeon the largest area of access that you can, with the site of surgical action in the middle. Exactly how you do this will depend on which retractors you are using, and if any self-retaining instruments are being used. However, it is helpful to think of the shape of the 'hole' in which you are operating. For example, if you are holding a retractor in each hand, and the surgeon is retracting towards his or her own body, it is often helpful to arrange your retractors 120° apart from each other and from the surgeon's point of retraction. Together with the surgeon, you are then forming an approximately equilateral triangular wound opening. This gives the greatest surface area of exposure, and usually the best access and view (see Figure 6.2).

You will be able to give the surgeon the best assistance if you understand what he or she is trying to do. If you are unsure of what the surgeon is trying to achieve, and you feel that you are not helping the surgeon to the best of your ability, it is best simply to admit this, and ask.

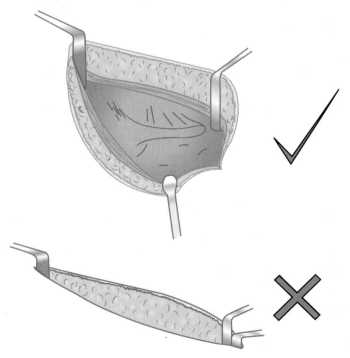

**Figure 6.2**   Top: the assistant is holding the two retractors (on the right of the illustration) well apart, at about 120°; this gives an approximately equilateral triangle, and the best surgical exposure. Bottom: the assistant's retractors are too close together, at a narrow angle, resulting in poor surgical exposure.

# 7 General stages common to operations

Most operations can be broken down into a series of stages. Not all operations contain every stage. These stages include the following.

## ■ Preparation by the anaesthetist

This includes such procedures as inserting intravascular cannulae, which may be intravenous (peripheral or central) or intra-arterial, placing monitoring electrodes and warming blankets, administering the anaesthetic itself (general, regional and/or local), endotracheal intubation, and administering other drugs that may be needed, such as heparin or prophylactic antibiotics. The number of these procedures needed varies greatly, depending on the patient's fitness and the type of operation. For a small operation in a fit patient, anaesthetic preparation may take under five minutes, while for a major operation in an unfit patient, it may take well over an hour.

Unfortunately, some surgeons resent this preparation time, as they feel their time is being wasted by the anaesthetist. In the author's (perhaps heretical) opinion, this resentment suggests an unprofessional lack of respect for colleagues. While the surgeon may feel, for example, that an arterial line is unnecessary, it is the anaesthetist who will have to contend with intra-operative hypotension should it arise.

## ■ Setting up (positioning the patient and equipment)

### Patient positioning

Anaesthesia, particularly general anaesthesia, renders the patient helpless and therefore dependent on the theatre staff to avoid injury. Space limitations do not allow a proper explanation here of the large number of different positions in which patients are placed for different operations. Several excellent textbooks have been written on this subject, and readers are referred to these (see 'Suggested further reading', p. 201).

However, the basic principles are to allow proper access to the surgical site and possible extensions of it, while avoiding harm to the patient. Usually, the patient should be secured in a position that looks as though it would be comfortable if the patient were not anaesthetised. Most operating theatres have a variety of equipment to help keep the patient in a secure position. This equipment includes the operating table itself, and accessories that can be easily clamped onto it such as padded poles, limb-holding gutters and stirrups. Other equipment includes simple pillows, and specially-shaped bolsters and gel pads, all of which are sometimes held in place by careful taping with sturdy adhesive tape.

Tissues that should be protected by proper patient positioning include:

1 *Skin*: Avoid pressure against hard objects, such as retractor-poles, by placing soft gel pads appropriately. Prevent the patient's skin from making contact with metal objects, to avoid the possibility of diathermy burns. Patients with fragile skin, such as the elderly, need to be positioned with particular care. For example, adhesive tape used to secure padding should not make contact with the patient's skin. This is because the tape may tear the skin when it is removed at the end of the operation.

2 *Nerves*: Avoid excessive traction (e.g. on the brachial plexus, by not abducting the shoulder to more than 90°) and direct pressure (e.g. on the ulnar nerve at the elbow, the common peroneal nerve at the knee).

3 *Musculotendinous structures*: Be careful when positioning the limbs of an anaesthetised patient. Because protective reflexes are reduced or absent, limbs can easily flop around excessively causing injury. For example, if you move the leg by grasping only the foot, with the knee flexed, gravity can cause sudden unrestrained full extension at the knee, causing meniscal or ligamentous injury to the knee.

## Applying anti-thromboembolic devices

These include stockings and calf compression devices. The stockings superficially resemble women's white dress stockings, but are much tighter fitting on the legs. This is because they are woven with elastic, so that they squeeze the legs, compressing the deep veins. This decreases the likelihood of clot developing in the veins, to form a deep vein thrombosis (DVT).

Calf compressors are usually pneumatic. They intermittently inflate, squeezing the legs and helping to prevent blood pooling in the deep veins.

### Shaving

Sometimes this is done prior to arrival at the operating theatre. It is discussed in more detail on p. 45.

### Skin preparation

This term (often abbreviated to 'prep') means the act of painting the skin with antiseptic solution. It is also used for the solution itself (see also p. 45).

### Draping

This means placing sterile sheets around the surgical site (see p. 47).

## ■ Marking the incision with a surgical skin-marking pen

For most operations using a standard linear incision, this step is unnecessary and is omitted. However, skin marking is a very important part of some other operations. In particular, in operations where skin is excised (rather than merely incised), skilful pre-operative planning and skin marking will determine not only the final appearance, but also sometimes, even whether the skin wound can be closed at all. Examples of this include mastectomy for cancer, and many plastic surgical operations.

## ■ Entry

Incision of the skin and other tissues overlying the operative site, such as fat, muscle, fascia and bone.

## ■ Mobilisation

This is the process of freeing up of the organ of interest, from surrounding structures.

# ■ The key therapeutic objective

This is sometimes known as 'the tricky bit'. It may consist of:

Incision (e.g. drainage of an abscess).

Excision:

    1  as an investigation (e.g. lymph node biopsy); or

    2  as a definitive treatment (e.g. cholecystectomy).

Evacuation (e.g. of a subdural haematoma).

Exploration (e.g. of a traumatic wound).

Manipulation (e.g. antireflux surgery, coronary artery bypass grafting with internal thoracic artery).

Implantation:

    1  of prosthetic material (e.g. repair of an abdominal aortic aneurysm, hip replacement).

    2  of donor tissue (transplant).

# ■ Reconstruction

For example complex musculofascial flap reconstruction after excision of cancer of the upper airway; anastomosis of the terminal ileum to the transverse colon after right hemicolectomy.

# ■ Haemostasis ('stopping the bleeding')

In practice, this occurs intermittently throughout the operation. That is, the surgeon usually stops bleeding points soon after they are encountered. Many surgeons do a final check of haemostasis towards the end of the operation. The different techniques, and your role in them, are discussed on p. 52–3.

# ■ Washing out (also known as irrigation or lavage)

This means irrigating an area (often with normal saline) to remove small pieces of debris that may act as foreign bodies, or as a culture medium for infection. This debris may include loose fatty tissue, blood clot and fibrin.

# ■ Drain insertion

Not all operations contain this stage.

## ■ Closure of the wound

Some or all of the layers of the wound ae closed. Most commonly, the layers are stitched closed with suture material. Occasionally, other methods are used – for example, a hernial defect may be closed with plastic material, or the skin may be closed with staples.

## ■ Local anaesthetic instillation

This is usually done only for smaller wounds, to avoid potential problems with toxicity from large doses of local anaesthetic. Often, the local anaesthetic is injected at the start of the operation – and obviously this is always so, when local anaesthetic is the only type of anaesthetic the patient is to receive.

## ■ Dressings

Numerous different types of dressings exist, and surgeons all have their own favourites. The basic function of all dressings is to protect the wound and help provide an environment tha promotes wound healing.

## ■ Other: key points

As well as the general stages mentioned above, most operations have one or more key points, sometimes referred to as danger points or pitfalls. These often mean avoiding injury to important structures near the one being operated on. Examples include:

In thyroidectomy, avoid injury to the recurrent laryngeal nerve, and the external branch of the superior laryngeal nerve.

In cholecystectomy, avoid injury to the bile duct.

In right hemicolectomy, avoid injury to the ureters and duodenum.

In parotidectomy, avoid injury to the facial nerve and its branches.

If possible, aim to read up on these key points before the operation. They are an important feature of textbooks of operative surgery, that is usually absent from pure anatomy texts. Operative texts are generally better 'value for time' than anatomy texts if you are short of time, although in an ideal world, you would read both beforehand (see 'Suggested further reading, p. 201).

# Sterility and the 'sterile zone'

## 8

During an operation, certain sterile 'zones' exist in the operating theatre. These are usually centred around the operating table, and are easy to identify. For example, all the green or blue drapes are sterile. However, the exact outer borders of sterile zones are often surprisingly ill-defined (see 'where to put your hands', p. 42).

Most operating lights have a handle for the surgeon to adjust them; they are therefore provided with sterile over-handles, which may be either disposable plastic or re-usable metal or plastic. Some of them are screwed into place, while others (especially the disposable plastic type) are simply pushed firmly into place.

Unless you are scrubbed, gowned and gloved, do not enter the 'sterile zone'. For example, do not walk between two sterile areas (such as between the scrub nurse's trolley and the draped patient), and do not touch the drapes. If you accidentally breach the sterile field, it is essential that you admit your mistake. For example, if your gloved finger accidentally touches something unsterile when you are scrubbed, you must immediately stop using that hand in the sterile field (unless removing the hand will cause a problem), and request a new glove from the scrub nurse, as soon as the opportunity arises. No-one should think badly of you for doing this; on the contrary, they will probably be pleased with your honesty and respect for the sterile field.

Another common way that the sterile field is accidentally breached, especially if you are tall, is by brushing your head (or hat) against the sterile light handle. If only your hat touches the handle, you may not feel it. Therefore, if someone else tells you this has occurred, do not think he or she is persecuting you. It is possible that he or she may be wrong, and your hat only passed near the handle, without touching it. However, if there is any doubt, the handle should be replaced.

The degree to which a surgeon will adhere meticulously to sterility will vary according to the operation. Clearly, meticulous asepsis is much more important when implanting a new cardiac valve, than when draining a perianal abscess (see also, 'prosthetic materials', p. 90).

# ■ Waterproof gowns

Prior to scrubbing, decide if you need a waterproof gown or not. The reason for wearing one is that blood and other body fluids can soak through standard gowns made of cloth ('wet undies phenomenon'). This is uncomfortable, and theoretically an infection risk. Decide if the operation has a reasonable likelihood of wetting you with body fluids, for example caesarean sections and most laparotomies. If so, you have two options:

1  Wear a plastic apron under a standard cloth gown. This will protect your torso, but not your arms.

2  Wear a waterproof gown instead of a standard cloth gown. These are usually made of a paper-like material. Their advantage is that they protect your arms as well as your torso, but with the possible disadvantage that they are slightly warmer to wear, and sometimes uncomfortably so.

# ■ Scrubbing

This is the word that is used to describe the systematic hand-washing done immediately prior to an operation. Skin cannot be sterilised without destroying it. The scrub merely decreases the bacterial population on the skin, although it can do so approximately 50-fold (Grabsch *et al.*, 2004). There is no universal agreement as to which method of pre-operative hand-washing is the best. The methods described below are believed by the author to be satisfactory, but should be regarded only as guidelines. It is usually best (and certainly diplomatic) to follow your own hospital's policies; these will probably have been developed using recommendations provided by the manufacturers of the specific hand-cleaning agents in use at that hospital.

## Scrub taps

Conventional bathroom taps are operated by handles, but this system is unsatisfactory for scrub taps, because the act of turning the (unsterile) tap off would immediately re-colonise the skin with bacteria. Therefore, surgical scrub taps are designed to be turned on and off without using the hands. Types include the simple mechanical foot-pedal or elbow-lever, and the electronic movement sensor, activated by moving the hands in front of a sensor. Simple mechanical taps have existed since ancient Roman times, and work perfectly well (Bruun, 1991). In the author's opinion, the same cannot always be said of the sensor types, which are sometimes prone to turn themselves on and off unpredictably.

## When to scrub

It is not always easy to know the best moment to scrub. If you scrub too early, you will be standing around with nothing to do. This can make you look foolish. It can also annoy some anaesthetists and scrub nurses, because some impatient surgeons deliberately scrub early to try to make them hurry! On the other hand, if you scrub too late you will not be ready to help the surgeon. Generally, the best time to scrub is at the same time as the surgeon, unless you are told otherwise. The scrub nurse normally scrubs well before the surgeon, to allow time to set up the sterile instruments. Therefore, you should almost never scrub before the scrub nurse, except in desperate emergencies.

## Scrub technique

The scrubbing sinks are usually just outside the operating theatre itself. Near the sinks will be several different antiseptics with which to scrub. These will usually include povidone–iodine-based preparations (e.g. 'Betadine®'), and chlorhexidine. Your choice is a matter of individual preference, but chlorhexidine and alcohol is probably more effective than iodine in reducing bacterial counts on the hands (MMWR, 2002). The different antiseptics may be dispensed from a squirting bottle, or they may be in disposable plastic packages containing a sponge or brush impregnated with the antiseptic. Scrubbing with a brush should probably be avoided, as it can damage the skin and cause increased bacterial shedding from the skin. A sponge is satisfactory.

Most single-use containers become slippery and very difficult to open with wet hands, so ensure you open them before starting to wash. Some theatres also provide mild soap, for people who are sensitive to chlorhexidine and iodine. However, soap is much less effective as an antiseptic, so use it only as a last resort.

Turn on the taps, and scrub the lather from your fingertips to your elbows. Always keep your fingertips raised higher than your elbows, to stop drips from running down to the fingertips. Clean under your fingernails, using a nail cleaner if one is provided. Otherwise, use the brush part of the scrubbing pad. Imagine the hands to be a series of planes, and scrub the whole of each plane systematically. For example, scrub your left hand first: scrub the palmar surface, including fingers, then the dorsum, then the medial edge, then between each of the fingers, then up over the thumb, then the fingernails. Repeat this for the right hand, and then repeat it for each hand. The duration of scrub varies according to different hospitals' policy, but a common regimen is 5 min for the first scrub of the day, with 3 min for each subsequent scrub.

## ■ Drying the hands

You do not dry your hands at the sink. Instead, rinse off the soapsuds, turn off the tap and walk to the gowns; sterile hand-towels should await you there. If not, wait until they are brought to you. Dry your hands in a systematic way, using a new area of the hand-towel for each part of the hand and then fore-arm. This is done because your fingertips are considered 'more sterile' (if there is such a thing as degrees of sterility) than your elbows. Dry each finger first, then your hands, then your fore-arms down to the elbows, and then discard the towel without bringing it back up to your hands.

## ■ Gowning

Next, put on your gown. The entire gown is sterile, but obviously, once you touch it this is no longer so. Therefore, it is important only ever to touch the inner surface of the gown, to keep the outer surface sterile. Unless you are certain that you will be using the 'assisted' method of donning your gloves (see below), do not push your arms all the way into the sleeves. Rather, push your hands into the sleeves only until they reach the narrow, elasticated wrist part. This is to enable you to don your gloves properly.

Once donned, surgical gowns are tied at the back with tapes; someone else (usually a scout nurse) will do this for you. This will usually be done for you while you are donning your gloves. This means that while your front is now sterile, your back is still unsterile. This situation is improved by the procedure known as 'turning your gown'. Two spare tapes, tied loosely together, are at the side or front of your gown, approximately at waist level. One is connected to a back flap, which will cover your back with sterile cloth. After you have donned your gloves, you grasp one of these tapes, and give the other to another scrubbed member of the surgical team to hold. You then turn a little pirouette, which brings the back flap across your back. Pause for a moment before doing this pirouette, and look at the gown to ensure that you will turn in the right direction to bring the flap across your back. Take the second tape back from whoever was holding it, and tie the two tapes together in front of you, or at the side. If the other person has not yet turned his or her gown, offer to return the favour by holding his or her tape. It is polite to do this before tying your own tapes together, so the other person is not kept waiting.

Instead of having the two tapes tied loosely together, some gowns (especially disposable gowns) have the two tapes attached to a playing-card sized piece of cardboard. This offers the slight advantage that the second person with whom you turn your gown, does not need to be scrubbed. This person holds the cardboard while you turn, and then you pull the tape out of the cardboard.

# ■ Gloving

## Glove size

If you do not know your glove size, say so. Average men's gloves are size 7½, while average women's 6½. If in doubt, it is better to wear them slightly too small, because otherwise the fingertips may be too loose. They will then flop around and reduce your dexterity. Many authorities recommend that two pairs of gloves be used routinely, to reduce the risk of disease transmission (see 'needle-stick injury', p. 9). This is known as double-gloving, and there is strong scientific evidence to support the practice (Tanner and Parkinson, 2002).

It is part of the set of procedures known as Universal Precautions (see p. 9). Despite the aforementioned recommendations, at the time of writing, double-gloving is far from universal.

If you wear two pairs of gloves, you may want to try combinations of different sizes. For some mysterious reason, they often seem to fit better with the larger size on the inside. For example, if you normally wear size 7½ gloves, you may find that wearing a pair of size 8 gloves underneath them is more comfortable than wearing the size 8s on the outside.

## Glove type

Standard surgical gloves are made of moulded latex rubber, and are disposable. They come in pairs which are usually marked 'left' and 'right' or 'L' and 'R', on the wrist. It is surprisingly easy to put a glove on the wrong hand. For a short operation, this does not matter much, but for a long operation, you will become uncomfortable as the glove presses your thumb posteriorly.

Some patients and staff are allergic to latex, in which case latex-free gloves (typically made of neoprene) are available.

To make them easier to put on, some gloves have powder on them to act as a lubricant. It is a common misconception that the powder is talc, but talc has seldom been used for this purpose since the 1950s. This is because it can cause severe inflammation in the tissues, which in the abdomen may lead to adhesion formation. Instead, the powder is usually cornstarch or calcium carbonate, which cause fewer problems than talc, probably because they are absorbable. However, it has been shown that these powders can also cause inflammation and other problems, both for the patient and for the wearer of the gloves.

Glove powder can act as a vehicle to transfer latex proteins, increasing the likelihood of latex allergy arising. It can also act as a vehicle for micro-organisms.

Therefore, most theatres now prefer powderless gloves. These are just as easy to don as powdered gloves, provided you dry your hands thoroughly first. If your hands are still wet, the gloves will not slide on properly, especially over your fingers.

## ■ Donning gloves

Gloves are put on after the gown. There are many different techniques for donning gloves. Broadly, they can be categorised into methods that require a scrubbed assistant, and those which do not. The unassisted methods are more common. They mean that you are not dependent on someone else to help you don your gloves, so it is essential that you learn one. The method described below is simply one of many. You may prefer to learn a local technique at your hospital, under the supervision of an experienced nurse or other staff member. The key point is not to touch the external surface of the glove with your bare hand or any other unsterile surface.

## ■ Donning gloves: unassisted method (see Figure 8.1)

Most sterile gloves are provided packaged in two layers of paper; an inner layer, which is sterile, and an outer layer, which is not. The outer layer is removed without touching the inner layer (usually by the scout nurse). The sterile inner layer containing the gloves, is then placed on a sterile surface (usually a trolley on which the gowns are also placed).

To don your gloves without assistance, you must obviously handle them. But the gloves are sterile, and your hands are not. How then, are you to handle the gloves without contaminating them? The answer is that to begin with, you only handle the gloves through your gown sleeve. You achieve this by ensuring that as you don your gown, you only push your hands into the sleeves as far as the narrow, elasticated wrist part (see p. 38).

Begin by unfolding the paper without touching the gloves themselves. This exposes the wrists of the gloves. The wrists are packaged folded back like trouser-cuffs, so that the inner surface (which will be in contact with your skin) is exposed.

Don the left glove first. Remove the glove from its pocket in the paper wrapping. With your left thumb and index finger, grasp the edge of the folded glove. Then slide your fingers into the glove. To help do this, use your (gown-covered) right hand to grasp the cuff of the glove at the point indicated by the arrow in the diagram, and pull the glove on.

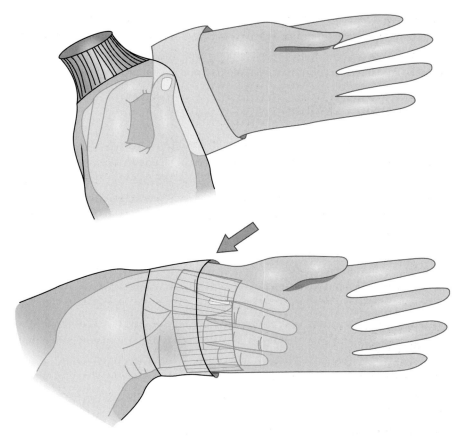

**Figure 8.1** Donning surgical gloves. The left hand is seen through the surgical gown's left sleeve. The left hand is inserted as shown, and the glove pulled on by gripping it with the right hand, at the point indicated by the arrow (see text, p. 40).

A variation of this method involves grasping the glove in the same way initially, but then placing the glove on the left sleeve of the gown, thumb downwards, with the fingers pointing towards the left elbow. The right hand is then used to flip the glove over while pushing the left hand into the glove, and pulling it on with the right hand.

You do not have to fit the glove perfectly at this stage; leave minor adjustments of the fingers for later. Now that your left hand is gloved, it is sterile. This means that putting on the right glove is easier, because you can handle the right glove with your left hand. Lift the right glove out of the paper with your left hand, and hold it open so you can push your right hand into it. Once both gloves are on, some final adjustments are usually necessary. For example, you will usually have to slide your fingers further in, to avoid having the fingertips of the gloves loose. Be careful that you do not touch the outer surfaces of the glove with your bare skin at any stage, because this obviously contaminates the glove with skin flora. If you do make a mistake, simply admit it, apologise, and ask for another pair of gloves.

## ■ Donning gloves: assisted method

Your assistant from this method will usually be the scrub nurse. He or she will hold the glove open at the wrist, and you simply push your hand into it.

Whichever method you use to don your gloves, ensure that the wrist of the glove makes contact with the cloth part of the gown's sleeve, not just with the soft elasticated part of the wrist. For some reason, if this is not done, the glove tends to slip off the gown, exposing an unsterile area of wrist skin (see Figure 8.2).

If you develop a hole in your glove, you must stop using the affected hand (immediately, unless doing so would cause a problem), and replace the glove. In this situation, the hand will often be wet (either from perspiration, or sometimes from the patient's body fluids that have entered the hole). In this case, ask the scrub nurse for something to dry your hand on, so that the glove is not too difficult to apply (see above section on 'donning gloves'). Similarly, if you notice that the surgeon or someone else has a holed glove, notify them immediately.

## ■ Where to put your hands (see Figure 8.3)

The precise borders of sterile zones are often surprisingly ill-defined. That is, while the clean operative wound is considered sterile, and the floor is obviously unsterile, there is an area in between which is neither. Arbitrarily, any area lower than the level of the operating table is usually considered suspect, even if it is covered by sterile drapes. This is important for two reasons. Firstly, you should keep your hands above this area. Secondly, if an instrument slips from the operating table, consideration should be given to replacing it, if it enters this area.

Similarly, some parts of a scrubbed person's surgical gown are not treated as sterile. By custom, only an approximately rectangular area on the front of the gown is regarded as being above microbial suspicion. Imagine a rectangle on your anterior torso, bounded superiorly by a horizontal line running through your mid-sternum, inferiorly by a horizontal line running through your umbilicus, and laterally by your anterior axillary lines. This imaginary rectangle is where you should rest your hands once you are gowned, gloved and waiting to take part in an operation (see Figure 8.3). It is comfortable to rest the hands together against the chest, as though praying but with fingers interlaced. Once sterile sheets have been placed on the operation site (see 'Draping', p. 47), you can step up to the operating table and rest your hands on it, until your help is needed.

It is surprisingly easy to become so engrossed in an operation, that you forget that there is a complete human being under the surgical drapes, and lean on him or her if you become tired. Do not do this. While it is acceptable and normal practice to rest

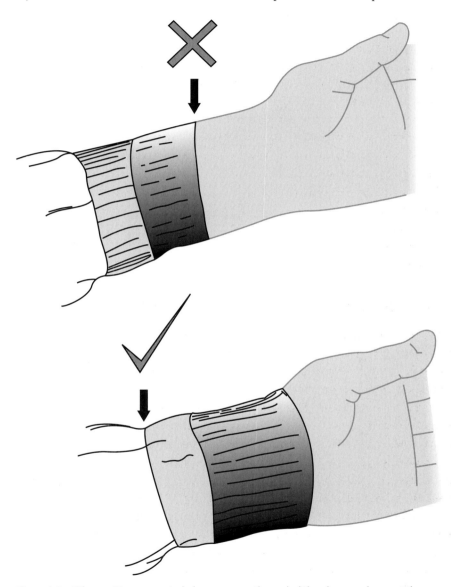

**Figure 8.2**   When putting on surgical gloves, ensure the end of the glove reaches past the elasticated wrist-band, giving plenty of contact with the cloth part of the gown.

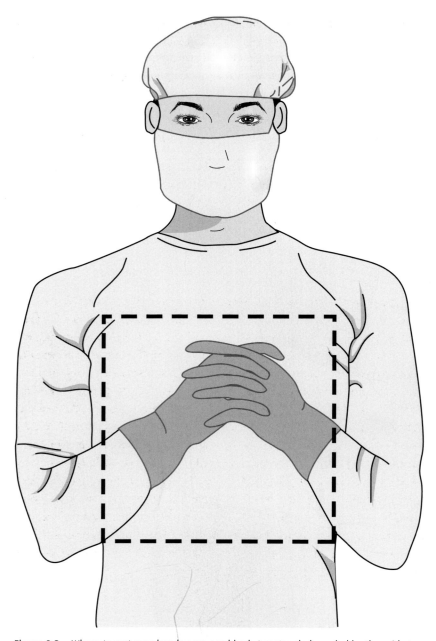

**Figure 8.3** Where to rest your hands once scrubbed. A rectangle bounded by the mid-sternum, umbilicus and anterior axillary line.

your hands lightly on the patient's body, leaning on the patient is potentially injurious. This is particularly so if the patient is a small child (see 'paediatric surgery', p. 145–6). If you think the patient would find your hands uncomfortable if he or she were awake, they should not be there while he or she is under anaesthetic.

# ■ Shaving, antiseptic painting and draping

There is a lot of individual variation in the way different surgeons will prepare the surgical field, even for the same operation. For this reason, the best thing to do is watch 'your' surgeon's method, and try to remember it for next time. However, the basic principles are as follows.

## Shaving

This is done because hairs harbour colonies of bacteria, and can easily become loose and fall into the wound. Electric clippers are better than blade razors, because blades cause tiny skin cuts that become colonised with bacteria. Different hospitals and surgeons have different protocols regarding shaving, but to decrease bacterial colonisation and consequent wound infections, it is best done within a few hours of the operation, or immediately beforehand (Alexander *et al.*, 1983). Some theatres supply small hand-held vacuum cleaners to remove the clipped hair. If one is not available, ask for some adhesive tape (e.g. 'Elastoplast'), stretch out 20 or 30 cm of it between your hands, and press it on the skin to remove the shaved hairs. Fine hairs, such as are typically found on a woman's abdomen, are not normally shaved.

Occasionally, a hair-bearing area will not be shaved. For example, in an extreme emergency, such as a patient who is haemodynamically unstable from intra-abdominal bleeding, omitting the shave saves vital seconds. The eyebrow is almost never shaved, because the resulting cosmetic defect is unsightly and because the eyebrow itself is a useful anatomical landmark to help close skin incisions precisely. Furthermore, facial wound infections are uncommon.

## Antiseptic painting

Antiseptic ('prep') is usually either povidone–iodine (e.g. Betadine®) or less commonly, chlorhexidine. As an assistant, you may be asked to paint it on. You will be given a small container of the antiseptic, plus an instrument with which to apply it. Most commonly, this will be a specially designed instrument (known as Rampley's sponge forceps), holding a piece of some absorbent material, such as foam rubber, in its jaws.

It looks more professional if you paint antiseptic on in a systematic way. There are many different and entirely satisfactory methods, although the author's preference is for the 'colouring in a shape' method:

1 Paint over the site of the intended incision itself (provided it is clean – see point No. 4, below). This gives the antiseptic more time to act against the local bacteria.

2 Mark out the area to paint (the 'shape' you will then colour in). Typically, a generous margin of about 15–30 cm in all directions is used. This may be even larger in some circumstances where the intended incision may need to be revised intra-operatively. For example, a surgeon painting the abdomen prior to an open appendicectomy (which normally needs only a thumb-length incision in the right lower abdomen) will often paint the whole abdomen, in case some unexpected pathology is encountered, and a midline laparotomy is needed. In other cases, the margin may need to be smaller, for example to avoid getting antiseptic solution in sensitive areas, such as the eyes.

3 'Colour in' the shape you have drawn. Using a second swab, start on the area where the incision will be made, and paint outwards in circles. Ensure you do not miss any small patches. Missed patches are especially likely to occur with some types of chlorhexidine, because it does not colour the skin in the same way as Betadine does. The same holds true when applying Betadine to patients with dark skin. In these circumstances, missed areas can sometimes be detected by carefully examining the glare reflected off the skin. Freshly prepped skin is wet and glossy; missed patches are dry and dull.

4 Paint potentially dirty skin crease areas (such as the umbilicus or groin) last, or preferably use a different sponge to paint them. Alternatively, dribble a little antiseptic in the umbilicus at the start of the paint, without touching it with the sponge. Otherwise, you risk contaminating the sponge with bacteria, and then painting them all over the operation site.

If the operation site is near a dirty area which could leak during the operation (e.g. a stoma), you will usually need to contain this before applying the antiseptic. Different surgeons have their own preferred methods of doing this, but typically, an absorbent pack is placed over the site, followed by an adhesive waterproof dressing (e.g. 'Opsite').

Some sensitive areas need to be protected from antiseptic. For example, cotton wool can be inserted into the external auditory meatus, and the eyes can be taped.

# Draping

Draping up (or towelling up) means to surround the site of the intended operation with sterile sheets, usually called drapes or towels. Like scrubs, they are usually green or blue in colour, because these colours are restful to the eye. The basic principle of draping is to cover most (and often all) of the patient's body with sterile sheets, while exposing the intended incision site with a small surrounding margin. Sometimes, local anatomical landmarks are also exposed, to help with orientation. For example, when draping up the right lower abdomen for an open appendicectomy, most surgeons will expose the anterior superior iliac spine and the umbilicus.

For some operations, the surgical field is draped symmetrically. Therefore, you can simply stand on the opposite side of the patient and mirror the surgeon's actions, just as you might if helping someone put clean sheets on a double bed. However, this will not always work, because for many operations, the drapes must be applied asymmetrically. Do not let the drapes touch the floor, or any other unsterile surface. If in doubt, simply ask the surgeon to instruct you.

Except for minor or dirty procedures, completed drapes usually have at least two layers of cloth. Sometimes this is done by simply using two sheets, but it is also done by folding a large sheet in two. In this case, the folded edge is usually placed at the border of the operative field. Often there is a waterproof sheet of plastic or paper between the layers.

At least one sheet may be raised to form a barrier between the operative field and the anaesthetist. This sheet serves several purposes. If the patient is awake (e.g. a patient having an operation under spinal anaesthetic) it spares him or her from watching the operation. It also helps to shield the anaesthetist from blood and other matter that may be projected from the operation site, and to prevent contamination of the surgical field by the unsterile anaesthetic field. It is sometimes known as the 'blood–brain barrier', a term that seems to enjoy greater popularity among anaesthetists than it does among surgeons.

## Clipping the drapes

The drapes are held in place with special instruments, unsurprisingly called towel clips. Occasionally, drapes are also sutured to the patient's skin to stop them slipping out of place during the operation. Some surgeons like to keep the towel clips out of the operative field. This gives a neater appearance, and more importantly prevents other things (such as suture material), from catching on the clips. This may be done by placing the clips under the drape, and then folding the drape back (see Figure 8.4(a, b). Alternatively, the clip may simply be flipped underneath the drape (see Figure 8.4(c)).

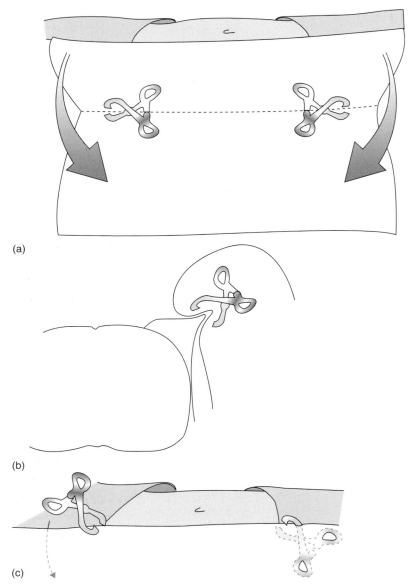

(a)

(b)

(c)

**Figure 8.4** How to conceal towel clips. In the first method (a, b), the towel clips are placed so that they grasp the first drape through the second drape. Note how the clips are placed away from the edge of the second drape, creating a flap, which is then folded (as shown by the dotted line) over the clips to conceal them. In the second method (c), no fold is needed. The first and second drapes are simply clipped together at their edges, and the clip tucked under the second drape to conceal it.

## ■ Setting up instruments

In all but the smallest operations, after the drapes are secured, some instruments will be placed in position before any incision is made.

For example, the diathermy pen or forceps, or both, will usually be placed in a tubular receptacle, known as a quiver, which is clipped to the drapes. Surgeons have their own preferences regarding where the diathermy quiver is positioned, so ask before clipping it. Typically, it is placed within easy reach of the surgeon's dominant hand. Place its electrical cord so that it will not get in the way of the operation. To prevent the cord becoming contaminated by falling directly from the quiver to the floor, a short length of it (perhaps 50 cm) is secured to the drapes. This is done by pinching up a small fold of drape-cloth, so making a little tunnel for the cord, and clipping the tunnel closed with a towel clip. Ensure that the surgeon has enough free length of cord to reach even the farthest reaches of the operation, but not so much that it will tangle and get in the way.

Hand the cord's plug end off the table, for one of the scout nurses or orderlies to plug into the diathermy machine. Avoid contaminating your glove by touching the nurse's unsterile hand. Do this by grasping the cord about 30 cm from the plug, and holding it out for him or her to take.

## ■ Incise drapes

In some operations, sterile self-adhesive sheets of soft clear plastic material, known as incise drapes, are placed on the draped operative field. Their purpose is to cover the exposed, antiseptic-treated skin completely with a sterile surface, before any incision is made. The skin is then incised through the incise drape (hence their name). Because skin is not sterile, even after proper painting with antiseptic, incise drapes are used in operations where sterile conditions are especially important. This includes operations where foreign material is implanted in the body, such as joint replacements, vascular surgery with prosthetic grafts, and hernia repairs using mesh.

Different proprietary brands of incise drapes include 'Opsite' and 'Ioban'. Depending on the size of the operative field, they may be as small as your hand, or as long as your leg. Although their size may vary, the principles of applying them do not. They are usually rectangular, with a smooth upper surface, and an adhesive lower surface, which is designed to stick to the skin and surrounding drapes. The adhesive surface has an attached peel-away sheet, rather like a 'Band-Aid' on a bigger scale. To make this peel-away sheet easier to remove, the free edges of it hang loosely from each end. The usual method of applying incise drapes is as follows.

The skin is painted with antiseptic in the usual way. Next, it is dried by mopping off excess antiseptic with a dry sterile pack, which is then discarded. The surgeon will stand on one side of the operative field, with you (the assistant) on the other. Each of you grasps two corners of the incise drape, holding it horizontally above the operative field. Hold the drape itself, but without holding the free edge of the peel-away sheet. This then allows the scrub nurse to pull the peel-away sheet off, leaving the adhesive surface exposed. Ensure you have a firm grasp, because if the incise drape slips out of your hand at this point, it will probably stick to itself in an irretrievable mess. Once the peel-away sheet is off, do not immediately lower the incise drape onto the operation site. Rather, watch the surgeon place his or her end of it onto the cloth drapes and smooth it into position. Only then lower your end carefully, while the surgeon progressively smoothes the incise drape onto the operative field, preventing air bubbles becoming trapped under it.

During the entire procedure, hold the incise drape under just enough tension to keep it taut, but without stretching. If it is stretched when it is applied to the operative site, it will tend to contract and spring free of the skin soon afterwards.

# Tissue planes: traction and counter-traction

## 9

Finding the correct tissue plane is a key to many operations. Anyone who has ever peeled an orange is already familiar with the concept of tissue planes. By pulling the peel in one direction, and the edible flesh in the other, the orange is peeled. In many parts of the body, a similar plane exists between two structures, which the surgeon aims to dissect apart. They are sometimes called avascular planes, but this name is not always accurate. While it is true that they frequently contain very few or no blood vessels, they often contain some small vessels, and occasionally quite large vessels.

Often, the correct tissue plane can be confirmed by the appearance of fine loose areolar tissue in the 'valley' between the two pieces of tissue being separated. This areolar tissue looks a little like spider-web, and is very delicate. It can easily be divided with the fingers, and sometimes is. It is often seen, for example, when mobilising the colon or duodenum from the posterior abdominal wall, when dissecting the breast off the thoracic wall, and between the muscular layers in an inguinal hernia repair.

Unfortunately, most tissue planes in the human body are more difficult to identify than in an orange. Sometimes, the planes may be partly or even completely obliterated. This obliteration has a number of causes, including malignancy and inflammation.

At the time of surgery, inflammation may be active, or it may have resolved ('burnt out'). It may be caused by the disease for which the operation is being done, or by previous surgery. Importantly, the effect of inflammation on the tissue planes varies, depending on how long it has been present. Two key characteristics of inflamed tissue are an increased blood supply and the presence of exuded fluid. While this fluid may sometimes help to define tissue planes, the increased vascularity makes the operation bloodier, so the net effect of inflammation on tissues is usually to make an operation more difficult.

Between the onset of acute inflammation and its resolution, there is an intermediate phase when the tissues become 'gummed up', adherent to each other, friable and bloody. Its time of onset is somewhere between 3 days and 1 week, and it continues for several weeks or months. Surgeons try to avoid operating in this phase whenever possible.

Even the most delicate surgery causes local trauma to the body, and therefore inflammation. This causes permanent disruption or obliteration of tissue planes to a variable degree. That is why 're-do' operations take longer, are more difficult and bloodier than 'primary' surgery, and are generally not enjoyed by surgeons.

If you can see the correct tissue plane, you will greatly help the surgeon by gently retracting the tissue on one side of it, while the surgeon grasps the tissue on the other side of the plane, retracts in the opposite direction and completes the dissection with the scissors, scalpel or diathermy. This technique is known as counter-traction. It must be done gently, to avoid tearing the tissues. Aim to retract with just enough tension so that, as the surgeon divides the tissue in the middle, the tissues on either side spring apart slightly (see Figure 9.1).

Counter-traction can be achieved by several different methods, mainly using instruments but occasionally the fingers. An example of the latter technique is

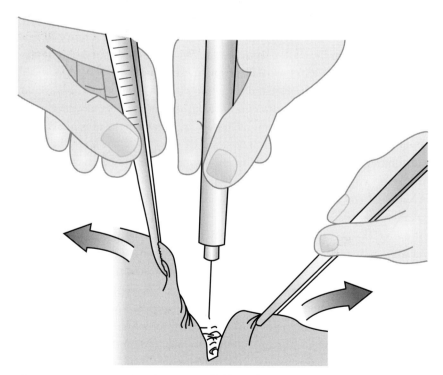

**Figure 9.1** Counter-traction. The assistant (left) gently retracts in the opposite direction to the surgeon, while the surgeon completes the dissection with diathermy.

sometimes used when opening the abdomen at laparotomy. When using this technique, the surgeon may ask you to place your fingers in the skin incision, and pull it towards yourself. A pack placed in the wound will help prevent your fingers from slipping. Sometimes the surgeon will simply want you to retract the fat towards yourself, while he or she completes the incision with the scalpel or diathermy. However, the fat here has a natural tendency to split along the midline. Some surgeons will exploit this natural splitting tendency by simply pulling the wound edge firmly towards themselves, once the skin is incised. This causes the fat to split down to the midpoint between the rectus muscles, which is the usual point of entry at laparotomy. If the surgeon is using this technique, it is important that you (the assistant) also pull firmly. Although the technique may look brutal, in the author's opinion it is less traumatic to the tissues than using sharp dissection, and delicately veering off into the incorrect plane.

Grasping instruments that are commonly used to provide counter-traction include forceps (e.g. De Bakey), and ratcheted grasping instruments such as Babcock's or Littlewood's forceps. Alternatively, gauze can be wrapped around your finger (because it does not slip on tissues like surgical gloves do), or wrapped in an instrument such as a sponge-holder (a 'swab-on-a-stick', see p. 82). For your own comfort and that of the surgeon, always keep your fingers away from sharp instruments. Occasionally it is useful to use a fine sucker (e.g. the Yankaeur sucker) as a retractor, because you can suck tissue fluid out of the way simultaneously.

# 10 Surgical instruments: their names and how to use them

## ■ Introduction

Some surgical instruments look similar to common household tools, such as scissors or tweezers. Although you may feel that you can already use such instruments skilfully, the way you hold and use them is almost certainly not the standard surgical method. It is important that you cultivate the habit of using the standard surgical grips described below. They are acknowledged to give the best control of the instruments. For this reason, surgeons themselves use them. Furthermore, using any other grip will immediately mark you out to the surgeon's eye, as a complete novice to the operating theatre.

Surgical instruments are made in a vast number of types. They frequently have eponymous names. The name usually distinguishes the basic pattern of the instrument, regardless of its size. Like other areas of medicine where eponymous names are used, the nice thing about the practice is that it reminds us of medicine's interesting history. The disadvantage is that an eponymous name gives us no information about the object concerned, other than giving credit to the person who first described it. Even then, that credit is sometimes misplaced. Furthermore, very similar or even identical instruments are often called different eponymous names by different staff. Nevertheless, it would be a duller world if all surgical instruments were named in some purely descriptive, standardised way.

It is sometimes reasonable to keep one or perhaps two frequently used instruments (e.g. suture scissors) either in your hand, or next to you on the drapes. However, it is bad practice to hoard instruments out of the scrub nurses reach, just in case you might need them later at some stage in the operation. Hoarding is bad practice for several reasons. Surgical instruments are precision-made, and even the cheapest are expensive compared to superficially similar items for home use. For example, a single pair of good quality dissecting scissors may cost several hundred pounds (or dollars). Hoarded instruments and their delicate working surfaces may be damaged by clashing together, or by falling off the operating table. Moreover, since the scrub nurse cannot clean the instruments promptly if they are hoarded, blood and small pieces of tissue will dry on the instruments making them work less well, and harder to clean. Finally, when you want a particular instrument, you must take your eye off the operation to find it and orient it correctly in your hand.

# ■ Types of surgical instruments

## Basic instruments

For convenience, the author has classified these into cutting instruments and gripping instruments.

## Cutting instruments

### Scalpels: Barron and standard handles

Most scalpels are in two parts: the blade itself, which is disposable, and a handle, which usually is not. The most commonly used handle is a simple flat design, which looks vaguely like, and is normally held in a similar way to, an ordinary dinner-knife handle. For finer work, a Barron handle may be used. This is hexagonal in cross-section, like a pencil, and is also held the same way as a pencil.

A wide variety of different-shaped blades is available. The most common are probably the 20-blade, which has a full rounded belly; the 15-blade, which is smaller and used for finer work and the 11-blade, which has a straight edge coming to a sharp point.

### Scissors (see Figure 10.1)

Surgical scissors are made in a very wide range of designs and sizes. They vary from long-handled instruments as long as your fore-arm, and useful for reaching into a deep cavity in complex pelvic surgery, to tiny delicate instruments used for microsurgery.

As an assistant, the most likely purpose for which you will need scissors, is to trim sutures after they have been placed in the wound. The best scissors to use are simply those you are given for the purpose by the scrub nurse. These will commonly be mid-sized, robust scissors such as Mayo or Ferguson type, although it is usual simply to refer to them as 'suture scissors'. While different pairs of scissors may look similar, there will be differences between them. Even if the scrub nurse has two pairs of identical scissors, ensure you only cut suture material with the pair that has been allocated to this purpose.

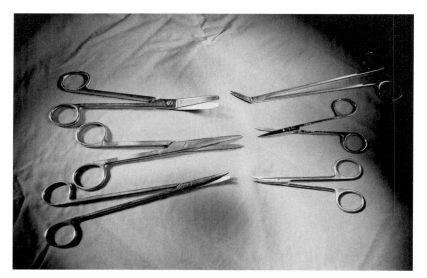

**Figure 10.1** Common scissors. Clockwise from top right: Pott's vascular, Iris, Tenotomy, Metzenbaum, Mayo, Ferguson's.

Slender scissor types such as Metzenbaum's are used for tissue dissection, and you will blunt them, and possibly damage them, by using them on something tough like suture material. You will also make yourself unpopular with the scrub nurse, which is a bad start to your surgical career.

An easy way to remember the names of Metzenbaum and Mayo scissors, is that the Metzenbaum's are long and slender like the written word 'Metzenbaum', while Mayo scissors are short and fat, like the written word 'Mayo'.

### The correct scissor grip

Refer to Figure 10.2. Because scissors have finger-sized holes in the handle, it is easy to think that the fingers should be inserted right through them. However, this is not necessary, and indeed, tends to make them more awkward to handle. Notice how the ring finger, thumb and index finger form a triangle, which from an engineering viewpoint is a rigid, stable structure. This gives precise control of the instrument.

Whenever possible, stabilise the scissor blades by resting them on something else, ideally the index finger of your opposite hand.

Cut with the tips of the scissors, not the main part of the blades (see Figure 10.3). This is for three reasons. Firstly, the tips are usually the sharpest part of the blades. Secondly, if you cut with the mid-part of the blades, it is possible that the tips will also inadvertently cut something else, perhaps the sort of something that should not be cut. Thirdly, you will have better control.

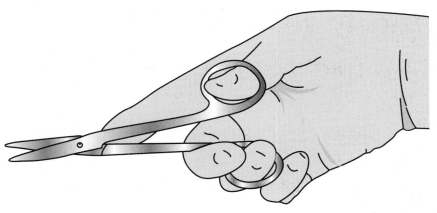

**Figure 10.2** Correct scissor grip. The thumb rests in one ring of the scissors, the ring finger in the other, while the index finger rests well down the blades. Therefore, the index finger, thumb and ring finger together form a triangle, a stable structure.

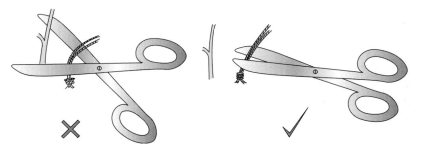

**Figure 10.3** Cutting with tips of scissors. Note how cutting with the tips avoids injury to the important structure at left.

*Cutting sutures*

Good scissors, used correctly, will cut through most suture material with a single cut. If they do not, sometimes you can improve their cutting ability by holding them at an angle of approximately 45° to the suture material (Figure 10.4). If the scissors still cut poorly, and especially if you find they are chewing their way through suture material rather than cutting, they may be blunt. To prove the point, and perhaps to prove that you are not 'a bad workman blaming his tools', you may ask someone else (e.g. the scrub nurse) to try to cut with them. It helps to accompany this request with a self-effacing remark like:

'I can't seem to cut with these. I'm not sure if it's me or the scissors. Do you mind trying them?'

If you have been using the scissors in the way described above, you will almost always find that the second person cannot cut with them either, and the scrub nurse will send them off for sharpening or repair.

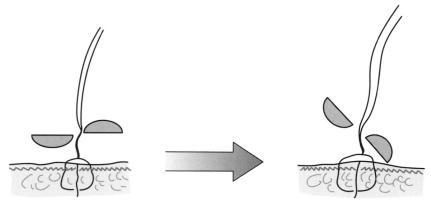

**Figure 10.4** Angling scissors to improve the cut. (The scissor blades are viewed end-on.) Angling the blades can improve their cutting ability.

Always cut the sutures to the correct length. That advice is very easy to write, but difficult to abide by. A standard joke in the operating theatre is: 'There are only two ways to cut sutures for a surgeon; too long and too short.' As a guide, when cutting interrupted sutures, cut them to a length that is similar to the space between each suture. This ensures that the cut end is short enough that it will not get in the way during tying of the next suture, but long enough not to let the knot unravel (see Figure 10.5).

For sutures other than interrupted type, it can be more difficult to judge how long to cut the free ends. Generally, it is better to cut slightly longer for monofila-ment suture material (which is the sort that looks like fishing line), and shorter for braided suture material (the sort that looks like shoe-laces). This is because monofilament suture material tends to slip on itself, and therefore has a greater tendency to allow knots to unravel, than does braided suture material. However, if you are unsure how long to cut a suture, the simplest and best method is prob-ably just to place the scissors about 4 mm above the knot, ready to cut, and then check with the surgeon if that distance is correct before cutting.

Ensure a suture is cut completely through before pulling the scissors away. This may seem obvious, but it is important because often when a suture is not cut completely through, the suture material gets stuck between the closed scis-sor blades (see Figure 10.6). In this situation, hastily pulling the scissors away will also pull the suture material, and is likely to tear the attached tissue. To avoid this, pause for an instant before removing the scissors. Once you can see that the suture is divided, you can remove your hands quickly.

Another situation where it is important to cut sutures to the correct length, arises when the suture is used not to hold the tissues together, but instead as a convenient

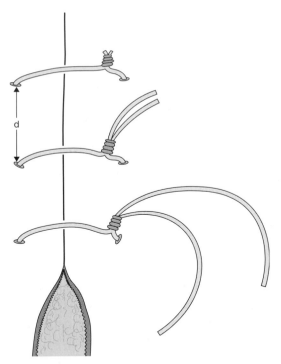

**Figure 10.5** Correct length to trim interrupted sutures. The top suture has been cut too short, which may allow the knot to unravel. The bottom suture has been cut too long, and the free ends may interfere with placement of subsequent sutures. The middle suture is correct: about the same length as the distance ('d') between each suture.

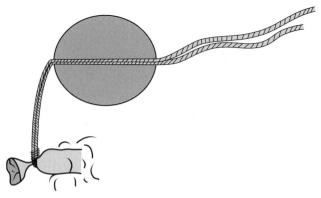

**Figure 10.6** Suture material caught between the scissor blades. (The scissor blades are viewed end-on.) Pulling the scissors away in this situation, can easily tear the ligated blood vessel.

way of marking an excised piece of tissue, to help orient it for the pathologist. This technique is commonly used in cancer surgery, especially surgery for breast cancer and skin cancer. That is, in most cancer surgery, the cancerous lump is removed with a surrounding margin of normal healthy tissue, to minimise the chances of leaving any cancer in the patient. The pathologist will examine the margins of the specimen histologically to ensure they do not contain cancer. If the margins do contain cancer, this is often an important determinant of future treatment for the patient. For example, another operation may be needed to remove more tissue from the area neighbouring the involved margin. In such a situation, it is obviously vital to know just which part of the wound should be re-excised.

However, once a piece of tissue is excised from the body, it is not always obvious 'which way is up' on that piece of tissue, because it may not have any anatomical clues on it. The problem is often solved by simply marking the specimen with suture material. A common method involves inserting sutures of different lengths on different margins, according to the system: 'Short is Superior, Long is Lateral, Medium is Medial'. Using this system, the exact length of the suture material is unimportant, provided that the different lengths are easy to tell apart, and that the short suture is not so short that it is hard for the pathologist to find, or worse still, falls out.

Each time a suture is trimmed, a scrap of suture material results. If you have a spare hand and can do so unobtrusively, remove these scraps from the operative field. It is best to pass them to the scrub nurse for disposal. Leaving them in the operative field allows them to get in the way of the operation, or stay in the wound as unnecessary foreign bodies. Throwing them on the floor is untidy and unpopular with the theatre staff, because they have to clean them up afterwards.

### Placing clips on sutures

Artery clips are placed on the end of sutures for several reasons. These include: to allow the suture to act as a retractor; to mark a particular anatomical point (e.g. the mid-point of an anastomosis); to stop the free end of the suture from being pulled all the way through the tissue being sewn, or simply to keep the free end out of the way.

Placing an artery clip on a piece of suture material is clearly quite a simple task. However, even simple tasks can sometimes be done in ways that are better or worse, and this task is an example. The clips will grip better if the jaws are placed at an oblique angle (perhaps 45°) to the suture material, rather than perpendicular to it. This is because the jaws usually have transverse teeth, so suture material placed exactly transversely can slip out between them, like dental floss between human teeth. This is particularly so with fine monofilament suture material (e.g. 4/0 nylon or polypropylene).

Usually the surgeon will indicate where he or she wants the clip to be applied before it is cut, but if not, try to apply the 'middle ground' principle (see 'medio tutissimus ibis', p. 5). That is, allow the surgeon enough suture material to work with (e.g. to hand-tie knots with), but not so much that suture material is wasted. Fifteen to twenty centimetres are usually about right.

*To cut or to clip?*

Most surgeons will tell you whether they want a suture to be cut or clipped. They will hold it up and say, 'Cut' or 'Clip'. However, some will simply hold a suture aloft with a silent air of expectation. In this situation, you are expected to know automatically whether you are supposed to cut it, or place an artery clip on the end of it. If a suture is being held aloft with this silent air of expectation, some- times the posture of the surgeon's hand will give a clue. If the end of the suture is clearly being proffered to you, this is probably a request for a clip. If not, and you are uncertain whether the suture is to be cut or clipped, ask the surgeon.

*Handling multiple clipped sutures*

In some operations, a dozen or more free ends of suture material may be clipped sequentially, for later tying (e.g. suturing in an artificial cardiac valve, or joining small bowel to the bile duct ('biliary-enteric anastomosis')). The reason for delay- ing the tying, is that it is easier to place interrupted sutures when there is easy access to both sides of the objects being sutured. That is, if each suture is tied as it is inserted, this obviously brings the two objects close together, making it harder to place subsequent sutures. Instead, when two objects are being sutured together with multiple interrupted sutures, it is often easier to place the sutures accurately if the objects are held a few centimetres apart. Once a suture is placed, its two ends are clipped together without tying. After all the sutures have been placed satisfac- torily, the two objects are then brought together, and all the sutures tied sequen- tially. Often the two objects are brought together by gently lifting the sutures taught, and sliding one object down to the other along them. This technique is known as 'parachuting', because of the resemblance of the multiple taught sutures to the suspension lines of a parachute (see Figure 10.7, and also 'vascular surgery', p. 177).

Sometimes, a large number of clipped free ends of suture material are formed. These clips, with their attached suture material, can easily become tangled together. To avoid this, as each clip is applied, thread a finger-ring of the clip sequentially onto a closed single long clamp, such as a Black's (see Figure 10.8).

A related technique is sometimes used when preparing a tie-over dressing for a skin graft. Here, after a skin graft has been placed in a wound, the edges of the

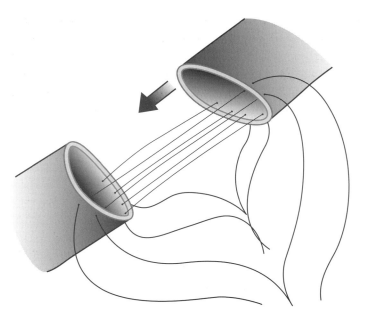

**Figure 10.7** 'Parachuting' two tubular structures together: a manoeuvre used in several different surgical subspecialties including cardiothoracic surgery, general surgery (especially colorectal and hepatobiliary surgery) and vascular surgery.

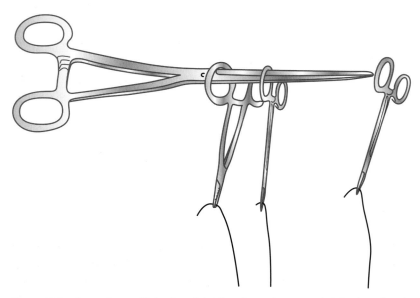

**Figure 10.8** Preventing multiple clipped ties from becoming entangled, by threading them onto the jaws of a long clip.

graft are sutured to the surrounding healthy skin, and the suture is tied in the usual way. However, instead of simply trimming both free ends of the suture material to 4 mm or so in length, only one end is cut to that length. The other end is cut longer (typically 10–15 cm) so that it can later be used to hold the dressing in place. To prevent these lengths from tangling, each free end can be clipped radially to the surrounding drapes, like the outer ends of the spokes of a wheel.

## Gripping instruments

These instruments are used for holding on to tissues. Broadly speaking, the better they grip, the more traumatic they are to the tissue. If a piece of tissue is to be removed during the operation, it usually does not matter much if it is somewhat damaged by a grasping instrument. Exceptions to this rule include situations where the damage may interfere with accurate histological assessment (e.g. biopsies for lymphoma), and where the structure to be grasped contains material that could be harmful were it to rupture (e.g. bowel contents, pus or tumour).

Some gripping instruments are sometimes described as 'atraumatic'. At the risk of being pedantic, it must be stated that few or no surgical grasping instruments are entirely atraumatic to the tissues. Perhaps it would be more accurate to describe them as 'less traumatic'. Such instruments are used for grasping delicate tissues, such as the bowel. Often, the degree of tissue trauma can be minimised by closing the jaws of the instruments only partially.

The extent to which most ratcheted instruments are closed can be conveniently measured in 'clicks'. That is, when a ratcheted instrument is closed slowly, the ratchet mechanism makes a clicking sound with each sequential slip of its small teeth over each other. For example, when atraumatic bowel clamps are placed on the bowel, the surgeon will sometimes state 'two clicks'; this is a request specifying the degree of gentle closure.

Unless directed otherwise, aim to close instruments with just enough pressure to hold securely, while minimising the crush effect.

### Ratcheted (see Figures 10.9 and 10.10)

*Atraumatic*

A Babcock grasper is a typical example of an atraumatic ratcheted grasping instrument. It can be used on delicate tissues, such as the bowel. Allis' forceps probably have a slightly more secure grip than do Babcock's, at the expense of slightly more injury to the tissues. They are used on tissues that are intermediate in sturdiness (e.g. breast tissue).

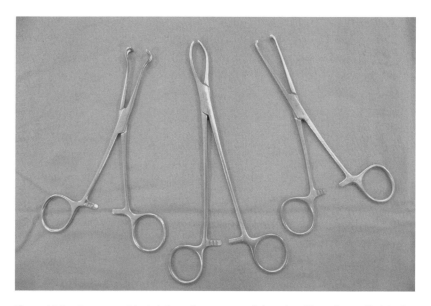

**Figure 10.9** Common ratcheted tissue forceps. From left: Babcock's, Littlewood's (also known as Rutherford Morison), Allis.

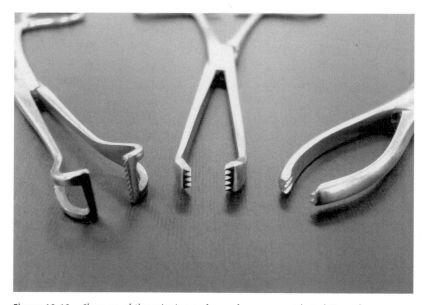

**Figure 10.10** Close-up of the gripping surfaces of common ratcheted tissue forceps. From left: Babcock's, Allis, Littlewood's.

*'Heavy'*

A Rutherford Morison (also known as a Littlewood's) has sharp interlocking teeth. It is useful for grasping tough fibrous tissue such as the rectus sheath, but will tear delicate tissues like the bowel.

*Clips*

Potential for confusion exists if the word 'clip' is used alone, as it could mean either an artery clip, or a small clip known as a Weck clip or Ligaclip. In some contexts, such as in vascular surgery, it could also mean a small clamp known as a bulldog clamp. These look vaguely like small metal clothes pegs. Artery clips are ratcheted instruments shaped vaguely like scissors, but with a ratchet mechanism (see Figure 10.11). Weck clips and Ligaclips are quite different to both of these instruments. They are small strips of metal (or sometimes another material) that look vaguely like standard office staples bent into a U-shape. They are used in some situations as an alternative to suture material, and are harmless when left in the body.

The U-shaped clip is mounted in the jaws of a special applicator instrument, with the limbs of the U pointing outwards. Closing the handles of the instrument closes the jaws, squeezing the clip. This closes the limbs of the U together, thus firmly grasping and compressing whatever is between them, rather like a ligature of suture material.

Weck or Ligaclips may be used to occlude small blood vessels, or other structures such as the cystic duct in cholecystectomy. The fact that metal Weck clips are radio-opaque means they are sometimes used as markers for X-rays. For example, when a breast cancer has been excised, Weck clips may be placed in the bed of the tumour, to help direct future radiotherapy.

*Types of ratcheted clips (see Figure 10.11)*

Larger varieties of these are sometimes called clamps. A wide variety of different eponymously named designs is available. The main points of difference between them are their size, the degree and type of angulation (if any), and the amount of crushing force they exert. When they are closed, most common clamps crush the tissue between their jaws. However, there are important exceptions to this, such as vascular clamps (see 'vascular surgery', p. 174) and the so-called 'soft bowel clamp' (see also p. 63). To prove the non-crushing nature of these instruments, surgeons (and assistants) will often apply them to their own fingers or web-space before applying them to the patient's tissues. A non-crushing clamp will cause no discomfort when this is done.

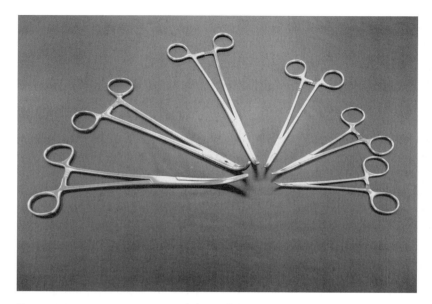

**Figure 10.11**  Some common surgical clips and clamps. From left: Roberts, Moynihan, Lahey, Mixter, plain artery, mosquito.

The commonest ratcheted clips are the so-called 'plain artery forceps' (also known as artery clips or haemostats). Mosquito clips are similar, but smaller and finer. Both of these clips may have straight or curved tips.

Common examples of angled clips include the Mixter, which has slender tips suitable for fine dissecting work, and the Lahey and Moynihan clamps, which are large, and mainly used for clamping major blood vessels prior to ligation. Surgeons may refer somewhat loosely to any of these angled clamps, as 'right-angles'.

### Non-ratcheted: forceps (never 'tweezers')

Many of these instruments look superficially like a larger version of household tweezers, but they are precision instruments (see Figures 10.12 and 10.13). A high degree of engineering skill is used in their manufacture, to ensure that the tips meet together in exactly the right way. Calling them 'tweezers' will instantly distinguish you as a novice in the operating theatre, so should be avoided. However, perhaps it would be better if these instruments *were* called tweezers, to avoid potential confusion with artery forceps. Still, this potential confusion only occurs occasionally, because there are many different types of forceps, used for different purposes, so a specific type is usually requested by name.

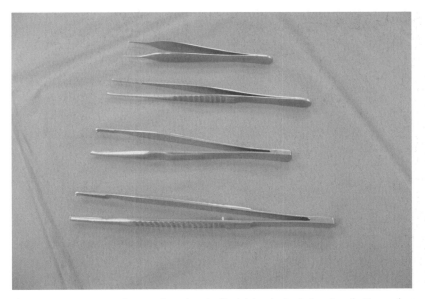

**Figure 10.12**   Common forceps. From top: toothed Adson's, De Bakey, Lane's, Bonney's.

Forceps may be broadly classified by whether they have sharp teeth at their tips (known as 'toothed forceps') or not ('non-toothed'). Unsurprisingly, they are available in different sizes.

Refer to Figures 10.12 and 10.13. Commonly used types of forceps include: toothed Adson's (fine forceps used for skin); Lane's (rather heavy toothed forceps used for tough fibrous tissue such as rectus sheath) and De Bakey's (medium-weight forceps with three interlocking rows of multiple fine teeth, originally designed for handling blood vessels, but also popular for general tissue work).

Always hold forceps like you would hold a pen, and not like a stapler (see Figure 10.14).

*Suture material*

As an assistant, you will almost never be required to choose suture material; that is the surgeon's responsibility. Therefore, a full discussion of the different types of suture material is beyond the scope of this text. Briefly, suture material is classified by several different properties. These include whether it is braided (like shoe-laces) or monofilament (like fishing line); whether the body absorbs it ('absorbable') or not ('non-absorbable'); whether it is made of synthetic material or naturally occurring fibres; whether it has a needle swaged onto it or not, and its thickness ('gauge', see Glossary).

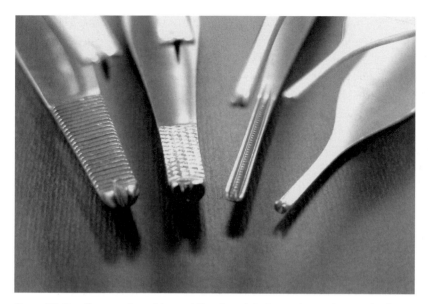

**Figure 10.13** Close-up view of forceps' tips. From left: Bonney's, Lane's, De Bakey's, toothed Adson's.

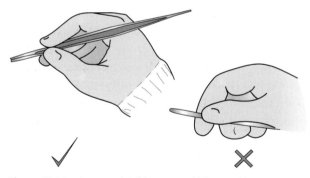

**Figure 10.14** Correct grip of forceps. Hold forceps like a pen, not like a stapler.

Modern suture materials are usually referred to by their trade name. Commonly used suture materials include 'Prolene' (polypropylene, a synthetic, non-absorbable monofilament); 'Vicryl' (polyglactic acid, a synthetic, absorbable, braided suture) and 'PDS' (polydioxanone, a synthetic, absorbable monofilament). Synthetic materials such as these have largely replaced older traditional materials like silk and catgut.

In the past, surgical needles resembled needles used in the home, in the sense that on one end was an eye, through which the suture material was threaded.

However, the threading was time-consuming, and the bulk of the eye and its double thickness of thread made a relatively large hole in the tissues. Today, virtually all surgical needles have no eye. Instead, the suture material is bonded (swaged) onto them by the manufacturer. Some suture material commonly used for ligatures (e.g. 'Vicryl') is also available for this purpose, without needles.

If you are required to handle suture material, avoid handling it with instruments unless expressly asked to do so. Grasping suture material with forceps, for example, will weaken it and make it prone to break. Although clips are often applied to the end of suture material (see p. 60), they are normally applied only to those parts of the suture that will be discarded.

*Suckers*

As their name implies, suckers are suction instruments attached to a vacuum apparatus. They are used to suck fluids away from the operative field. Suckers are also used to remove smoke made by the diathermy. They are metal or plastic tubes, with or without various embellishments. One end is attached to plastic tubing, which is connected to a reservoir. The evacuated fluid therefore passes into the reservoir, which has a capacity of a litre or more. It is usually made of plastic, and disposable. If the reservoir becomes full, the suction will stop working, and someone (usually a scout nurse) will change it.

Two major types of suction instrument exist (see Figure 10.15). They are:

1  *The sump sucker*: This is a tube about 15 mm in diameter, with rows of holes along it. It is used for sucking up large volumes of fluid quickly, for example irrigation fluid after washing out the peritoneal cavity ('lavage').

2  *Fine suckers (e.g. Yankaeur)*: These are used for delicate work. Most are simply a bent tube of metal or plastic with a handle on one end, and sometimes a rounded knob on the other end. The knob has several small holes in it, through which the fluid is sucked. Some have another hole higher up, in the handle. This lets in atmospheric air, therefore decreasing the strength of suction at the tip and making it more suitable for delicate work. The hole is designed to be occluded as needed by the finger or thumb, to increase the amount of suction at the tip.

Often both the sump sucker and fine types of suction instrument are used in one operation. This can be achieved in two ways:

1  Using a single piece of tubing and reservoir apparatus. Using this method, each time the different sucker is needed, the other one must be pulled out from the plastic tubing and replaced.

2  Using two sets of suction apparatus. This method is normally used only for large operations.

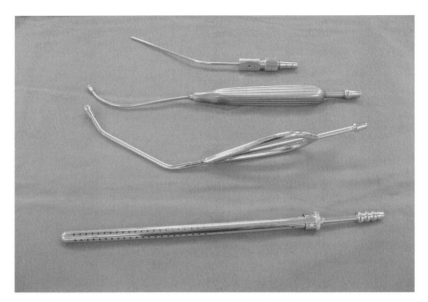

**Figure 10.15** Common suckers. From top: fine (McGucken), Paediatric, Yankauer, sump.

During operations, small amounts of blood and exuded tissue fluid tend to pool at the depths of the wound. When the surgeon is operating in those depths, you (the assistant) must remove this fluid, to ensure the surgeon can see what he or she is doing. It can be difficult to steer the correct middle course between sucking too much and not enough. Too much, and the sucker will clash against the surgeon's instruments and interfere with the operation. Not enough, and the fluid will pool and obscure the operating area. Sometimes, a skilful assistant can develop a rhythm with the operating surgeon, timing quick gentle dabs with the sucker so that they alternate with the surgeon's cuts: suck, cut, suck, cut (see Figure 10.16).

**If the sucker stops working**     Like most problems in life, it is usually best to try to fix it in a systematic way.

There are several different causes for the sucker stopping working. These include:

- The reservoir is full. A non-scrubbed member of the surgical team (usually a scout nurse) will change the reservoir.
- Debris is blocking the sucker or tubing. This can occur anywhere from the tip of the sucker to the reservoir. Examine the tip of the sucker, and dislodge any material you can see. If this does not solve the problem, ask the scrub nurse for a few hundred millilitres of saline. Immerse the tip of the sucker in the saline; this may dislodge the debris enough to fix the problem. If the sucker still does not work, pull the sucker out from the tubing. This will enable you to tell if the

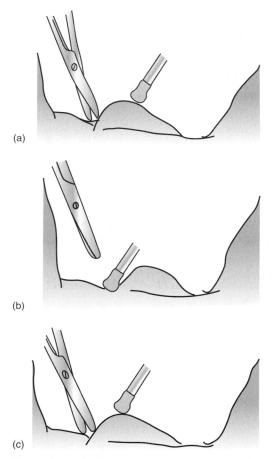

(a)

(b)

(c)

**Figure 10.16** As the surgeon dissects, keep the sucker poised nearby, ready to suck away accumulated fluid as soon as the surgeon lifts the scissors away.

problem is in the sucker, or in the tubing or beyond. That is, does the suction seem normal at the end of the tubing? (Can you hear it, and feel it with your finger over the end, and does it suck fluid up quickly?) If so, the sucker instrument is blocked and needs disassembly at some time. Depending on time availability, this may be done by you or the scrub nurse, or the sucker can be discarded and a replacement can be brought.

*Retractors*

As their name implies, retractors are instruments that retract tissues out of the way so that the surgeon can see what he or she is doing. As an assistant, you are very likely to find yourself holding one of these.

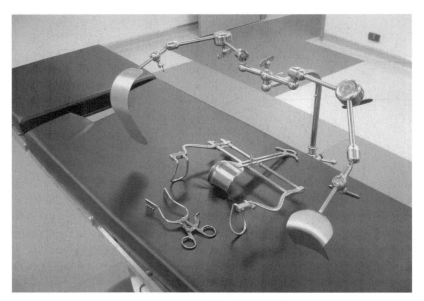

**Figure 10.17** Common self-retaining and table-mounted retractors. From left: Wietlander self-retainer, Balfour self-retainer (with third blade attached), Iron Intern (table mounted, showing two of the many different retracting blades available).

**Types of retractors** Retractors may be classified into two major types: those that hold themselves in place (see Figure 10.17), and those that must be held in place by the hand of the assistant or surgeon (see Figure 10.18). The self-supporting types may be attached to the operating table, or they may lie free in the wound. More accurately, these latter free-lying types usually hold themselves in place by the pressure they exert against the wound edges.

Broadly speaking, the table-mounted types are only necessary for major and complex cases, while the hand-held and free-lying types are used for smaller and intermediate-sized operations. The hand-held types may also be used in complex cases, to supplement the retraction provided by the table-mounted retractor.

The term 'self-retaining retractor' (often shortened to 'self-retainer') is in common use. Logically, it might seem reasonable to use this term to describe any retractor that does not need to be held in the hand. However, by custom the term is only used for the free-lying types, and not for the types that retain themselves in position by being attached to the operating table.

Hand-held retractors include the Langenbeck, Jackson, Morris and Deaver. The free-lying self-retaining type ('self-retainers') includes the Norfolk-Norwich, the Wietlander and the Balfour, while the table-mounted type includes the Bookwalter and the Iron Intern.

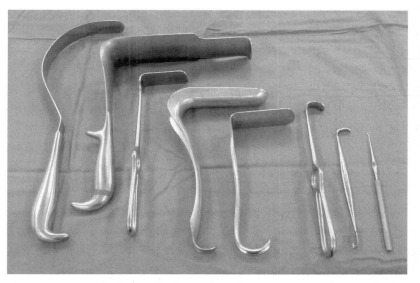

**Figure 10.18** Common hand-held retractors. From left: Deaver, St Mark's, Langenbeck, Sim's, Jackson, Kocher, cat's paw, skin hook.

**Hand-held retractors** Some hand-held retractors are fitted with comfortable ergonomic handles, while others are nothing more than a bent strip of metal, and can become quite uncomfortable on the assistant's hand. If you are required to grip one of these for long periods, you can sometimes minimise your discomfort by using two hands to spread the load, or adjusting your grip slightly at non-vital points of the operation. Of course, you could always ask for a more comfortable retractor. Sadly however, some surgeons have a cavalier disregard for the comfort of their junior staff, and if you are assisting such an individual, he or she may think you are 'soft'. In those circumstances, you may want to justify your request succinctly by saying something like 'I don't like to complain, but I think I could do a better job with a better retractor, if one were available.'

Hold the retractor by its handle. If it has no handle, grasp it comfortably close to one end. Do not allow your hand to creep down the shaft of the instrument so that you are holding it close to the lip. That is, as far as possible, ensure it is only the retractor that is in the wound, and not your hand as well. If your hand is in the wound, it may obstruct the surgeon's view, and expose you to the risk of a sharps injury.

Surgeons adjust retractors so that they expose the operative field in the most useful way. This applies both to self-retaining and hand-held types. Therefore, hold the retractor at the same angle and tension that the surgeon gives it to you. As a general rule, aim to keep the surgeon's operating instruments (i.e. scissors, forceps, etc.), especially their tips, free from impediment by surrounding tissues.

Retraction is easier if your hand or wrist is resting on something (usually the patient's body beneath the drapes) rather than being poised in mid-air. Remember, you may have to keep quite still in one position for long periods. Therefore, as far as possible, try to make sure that position is reasonably comfortable. However remember that, over-ridingly your role as an assistant is to give the surgeon the best view of the operation that you can, so be prepared to re-adjust your retraction appropriately (see also 'Improving the surgeon's view', p. 29).

It is especially important that the 'lip' of a retractor in the depths of the wound is kept still. Often the lip plays the most important part in tissue retraction (because it is closest to the action), but it can be the hardest part to see. Therefore, whenever possible try to see into the depths of the wound, when that is where the surgeon is operating. Obviously, this will also help you to follow and understand the operation better.

It is also important to ensure that the lip of the retractor is in the correct plane. Inexperienced assistants sometimes allow the retractor to slip out of the wound slightly, so that its lip is lying too superficially. When this occurs, the deeper tissue layers are free to interfere with the surgeon's actions. For example, an open appendicectomy wound is closed in layers, usually beginning with the peritoneum. At this point, retracting all the overlying musculofascial layers away from the peritoneum gives the surgeon the best access to close the peritoneum. Allowing just one of the overlying layers to lie free beneath the retractor's lip, will usually interfere greatly with this task.

Novice assistants sometimes pull very hard when retracting, perhaps in their enthusiasm to be helpful. However, this should be avoided whenever possible. When stretched, tissues often seem to behave a little like a rubber band. That is, a rubber band stretches easily up to a certain point, beyond which even a lot of force will stretch it only a little more, before breaking it. In the same way, retracting hard on tissues risks injuring them and does not usually give a great improvement in exposure. It is also tiring. If exposure of the operative site is inadequate, the surgeon will usually use some other manoeuvre, such as enlarging the incision, instead of hard retraction.

There are rare occasions when assistants are required to retract strongly. For example, when operating deep in the pelvis, it is usually not possible to improve access by enlarging the incision. (This is because in this situation, surgical access is limited by the narrow bony pelvis, and not by the skin and soft tissues.) It is often possible to make strong retraction easier by using your body weight instead of muscular effort, by leaning over slightly in the appropriate direction. This is much less tiring. Where possible, 'locking' joints straight, or bracing your elbows against your torso may also help. If you become tired, and feel that you are unable to continue holding the retractor or limb in its required position, tell the surgeon. Ask if it is possible to pause for a moment while you re-adjust your grip. While you may feel embarrassed by this, it is far better than continuing silently, then suddenly losing your grip while the surgeon is operating.

During the course of most operations, there will often be brief periods when your retraction is not needed. For example, the surgeon may pause briefly to change instruments. During these times, it is often beneficial to both the patient's tissues and your arms to relax your retraction, and then carefully resume it as the surgeon returns to the operative site.

Some types of retractors have sharp points on them, which if handled carelessly, can put holes in your gloves, and even in you. These include:

*'Cat's paw' retractors*: These look like a small Langenbeck retractor at one end, but at the other end, as the name suggests, is an array of hooks like a claw.

*Skin hooks*: These are fine retractors, used for retracting skin edges. They have a small sharp hook (about 4 mm across) which is driven into the skin.

**Self-retainers and table-mounted retractors**   These retractors are virtually always put in position and adjusted by the surgeon. However, you may be asked to help assemble and position some of the table-mounted types. There is a large variety of designs and it is beyond the scope of this text to describe them all in detail. The best plan is simply to ask an experienced staff member to help you as you learn the workings of your hospital's table-mounted retractors.

Broadly, most will arrive at the operating table complete, but disassembled, in a sterile tray on the scrub nurse's trolley. One or more sturdy anchoring poles are fastened securely to railings at the edge of the operating table, meaning that this part of the instrument is now unsterile. The next steps obviously depend on the design of the instrument, but often, sterile limbs are attached to these poles, and positioned near the wound. Lastly, retractor blades (which often closely resemble the blades of hand-held retractors) are secured to these limbs.

*Special equipment*

In many operations, highly specialised instruments are used, for example equipment for prosthetic joints, devices for stapling bowel together. Often these are designed for single use only. While the purpose and method of functioning of most surgical instruments such as scissors, forceps and retractors is obvious, this is often not the case with the more specialised instruments. Furthermore, because the surgeon usually uses these instruments at a key step of the operation (when he or she may not be in a communicative frame of mind), and then passes them off the table, it can seem difficult to learn more about them.

There are several ways to overcome this problem. In the packaging accompanying almost all single-use devices (e.g. surgical staplers), is a booklet provided by the manufacturer, describing the device in some detail. Usually, the surgeon and scrub nurse will already be very familiar with the device, and are unlikely to need this booklet. Therefore, to learn more about an individual device, you can simply ask the scrub nurse to keep the booklet for you, so you can read it after the operation. If you ask politely, most scrub nurses will also set the instrument aside for you to examine.

However, it is somewhat haphazard to learn about specialised instruments only when you encounter them at the time of an operation. Furthermore, it does not allow you to prepare for the operation in advance. Other sources of information include the theatre staff and surgeons, and some specialised texts (see, 'Suggested further reading', p. 201). Distributors and manufacturers of the instruments are usually very helpful, and willing to provide you with information about their products.

## ■ Diathermy

This instrument is used to cut through the tissues like a scalpel, and also to cauterise tissues to stop bleeding. It does both of these things by passing an electric current through the tissues, which causes intense local heating of the tissues at the tip of the instrument.

### Types of diathermy (see Figure 10.19)

The two basic types of diathermy are monopolar and bipolar diathermy. In bipolar diathermy, the electric current passes between the two blades of a pair of forceps, whereas in monopolar diathermy, the current flows from the forceps (or some other instrument), away through the patient's body to a special plate elsewhere on the skin.

Therefore, for bipolar diathermy to work effectively, the tissue to be diathermied must be between the forceps tips. The tips themselves must not be in direct contact with each other; otherwise, the current will simply flow from one tip to the other without much burning of the tissue. Bipolar diathermy is only used to stop bleeding, and almost never for cutting.

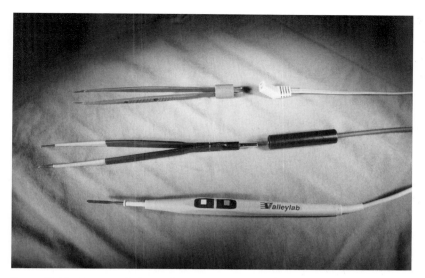

**Figure 10.19** Common diathermy instruments. From top: bipolar diathermy forceps, monopolar diathermy forceps, monopolar blade diathermy. The forceps have not been plugged into their leads, to show that the bipolar forceps has two electrodes, while the monopolar has only one. Note the two control buttons on the blade diathermy: one is for cutting and the other for coagulation.

In monopolar diathermy, the current passes between the operating instrument and a special conducting plate placed on the patient's body (usually on the thigh). Because this plate is large (slightly bigger than the sole of an average adult's foot), the current and heat at the plate is spread over a large area and does not cause a burn.

Whereas for bipolar diathermy the operating instrument is always a pair of forceps, for monopolar diathermy either a pair of forceps or a single blade may be used. The 'blade' may be a small flat strip of metal, or it may be a rounded wire terminating in a sharp spike or a round ball. One of these blades is mounted in an instrument that looks quite like a pen with a wire lead protruding from the end. The lead is plugged into a diathermy machine, which usually sits on a trolley next to the operating table. The blade diathermy is used both to cut and to stop bleeding, in contrast to forceps, which are normally used only to stop bleeding. To activate the diathermy, the surgeon presses either a foot pedal (for forceps diathermy), or a button mounted conveniently on the shaft of the blade diathermy 'pen'. Some makes of blade diathermy also have an attached tube, which is connected to vacuum apparatus, to suck out the smoke that the diathermy makes.

## 'Touching' with the diathermy (see Figure 10.20)

When the monopolar diathermy blade is in use, the surgeon may sometimes use a plain (i.e. non-diathermy) pair of forceps to grasp a vessel he or she wants to coagulate. A second person (usually you, the assistant) then completes the electrical circuit by placing the blade of the diathermy instrument against the surgeon's forceps, and activating the diathermy. This is known as 'touching' with the diathermy. Usually, a surgeon will ask you to do this by saying, 'Touch with the diathermy'. Sometimes they will say, 'Touch *me* with the diathermy', a request which should never be interpreted literally! Most pen-type diathermy units

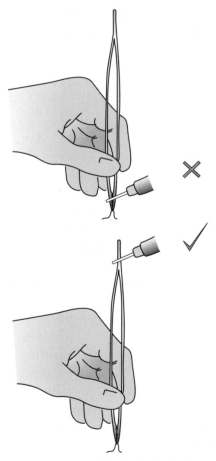

**Figure 10.20** 'Touching' with the diathermy. Top: Touching the surgeon's forceps below the hand obscures the surgeon's view and may dislodge the forceps. Bottom: The Correct method. Touch the diathermy above the surgeon's hand, near the top of the forceps.

are activated by pressing a button on the shaft. They usually have two control buttons: one for cutting and one for coagulation. Ensure you press the correct one. To avoid obstructing the surgeon's view, touch the blade near the top of forceps, not down near the tips. The diathermy machine will make a buzzing sound. It makes a different sound if the 'cutting' button is pressed.

Watch carefully so that you can buzz with the diathermy when the surgeon asks you ('asking' may take the form of a grunt); if in doubt, do not buzz. Ensure good electrical contact is made, but do not press the blade too firmly against the forceps, because this may tear their tips off the structure being held. Also, make sure the blade touches only the surgeon's forceps, and not something else (such as the patient's skin) beyond them as well. Keep the button depressed until asked to stop, or the surgeon lifts the forceps away. If the diathermy you are using does not have an attached smoke evacuator, and you have a free hand, use it to suck smoke out with the suction. This improves the view, and avoids inhaling the smoke. The risks of disease from smoke inhalation are probably small, but do exist. Regardless, the smoke smells unpleasant.

As an assistant, you may be asked to clean the diathermy blade or forceps. If you have a free hand, and can do so unobtrusively, you can also do this on your own initiative. The aim is simply to remove the deposits of carbonised material that accumulate on the instrument tips during the operation. There are two ways of doing this. The first is simply to rub the tips with another object, most usually a moist sterile pack. The second method uses a specially designed square of abrasive material, commonly known as a 'scratchy pad'. This is about the size of a large postage stamp, and has a self-adhesive backing to stick to the surgical drapes. The instrument is simply scraped against the pad. A combination of both the above cleaning methods usually gives the best results. Some diathermy blades are coated with Teflon to decrease the amount of carbon deposition; these can usually be cleaned by simply wiping them, without needing to use the scratchy pad.

## ■ Haemostatic techniques

### Overview

Haemostasis means simply 'stopping bleeding' (Greek haem means blood, stasis means stop). Intra-operative bleeding varies greatly in origin and rate, from very small vessels (so-called capillary bleeding) to frightening, audible, massive bleeding. Arterial bleeding is bright red and spurts, while venous bleeding is darker and usually wells up. If possible, try to avoid using the sucker to clear large volumes of active bleeding. It is better to apply pressure proximally to the source to minimise the bleeding, and only use the sucker to clear the remaining volume.

All surgeons use a similar array of techniques to control or prevent intra-operative bleeding. Obviously, different techniques are suitable for different rates of bleeding. In approximate order of increasing rates of bleeding, these techniques include:

1 Simply ignore it; it will stop by itself. Most 'capillary bleeding' (e.g. bleeding from the cut skin edge) is in this category
2 Diathermy
3 Clip and tie
4 Clip and double-tie
5 Suture
6 Transfixion-ligation

Other miscellaneous manoeuvres include:

- *Finger compression*: This is used both for very small bleeds (when it may be all that is needed) and for big bleeds (as a temporary measure to slow blood loss while its cause is fixed).
- *Topical application of haemostatic material (e.g. cellulose gauze)*: This is used for small volume oozing.
- *Argon plasma coagulation*: This is a special type of diathermy that uses argon gas. The gas emerges from the tip of the diathermy pen and conducts the current to the tissues like a miniature gaseous lightning rod. It is typically used in specialised situations to treat bleeding from large raw surface areas, such as the cut surface of the liver.
- *Ultrasonic shears*: This specialised instrument has a blade that oscillates at extremely high frequency (55 kHz). This vaporises the tissue, with minimal heating.

## Assisting with the different haemostatic techniques

### Simply ignore it

Obviously, the surgeon does not need any particular assistance for this technique, other than for you to ignore it too. This can sometimes create a minor dilemma in the mind of the assistant. That is, if you see a bleeding vessel, when do you inform the surgeon, and when do you leave it for the surgeon to attend to?

There is no simple answer to this question. However, generally, the correct answer is: 'If in doubt, tell the surgeon'. To help reduce doubt, ask yourself the following questions:

(a) Has the surgeon seen the bleeding? If he or she obviously has seen it, then it is better simply to wait for the surgeon to attend to it. Importantly, bleeding that may be obvious to the assistant's naked eye may not be obvious to a surgeon wearing loupes (magnifying spectacles), because these usually give a restricted field of vision.

(b) Is the surgeon currently attending to something more important?

(c) Is the bleeding likely to stop by itself (i.e. is it non-arterial and very small)?

Unless the bleeding is clearly so minor that it will stop by itself, or the bleeding is obvious and the surgeon is attending to some more urgent matter, it is better to inform the surgeon immediately.

## Diathermy (see also 'Touching with the diathermy')

### Dabbing

Often, you can help the surgeon to find the exact site of origin of a small bleed, by dabbing the area with absorbent material. This absorbs surrounding blood, so immediately after you remove the material, the bleeding source can be seen and diathermied. At other times, dabbing may be useful when the surgeon is doing something else nearby, because it prevents the blood from interfering with the surgeon's view. Sometimes the surgeon may ignore small bleeding points, while performing some other part of the operation. For example, blood often oozes from the cut bowel ends during a hand-sewn anastomosis, but surgeons will often ignore this because the volume is small, and may stop when the bleeding point is sutured as part of the anastomosis itself. Furthermore, most surgeons find such bleeding a pleasant sight, because it reassures them that their anastomosis has a good blood supply, and so is less likely to leak.

The key to using dabbing instruments is to ensure you dab, and not wipe, the tissues. Wiping simply encourages bleeding because it rubs off the small haemostatic plugs.

Dabbing instruments include the following.

*Gauze swabs*

These are pieces of loosely woven absorbent cloth. There are two commonly used sizes. The larger ones are about the size of a man's handkerchief, and are often simply called 'packs'. The smaller ones are about the size of the palm of an adult's hand. They usually have a thread of coloured radio-opaque material woven into the material. This is so they can be detected by X-ray, should they be inadvertently left in a wound. This is the explanation for their common name of 'Ray-tec' gauze.

*The 'peanut'*

This is a small piece of gauze, rolled up and mounted in the end of an artery clip or similar instrument. Its name arises from the fact that the rolled gauze is about the same size and shape as a peanut. Because the gauze is small, it can only absorb small amounts of blood, so the peanut is used for fine work.

*The swab-on-a-stick (also known as swab-on-a-holder)*
This is similar to a peanut, except both the clip and its contained gauze roll are larger. The gauze roll is about the same size as an average person's thumb.

Peanuts and swabs-on-sticks can also be used as dissecting instruments or retractors.

## Clip and tie

In this context, the verbs 'tie' and 'ligate' are used interchangeably. Once a surgeon has placed an artery clip on a bleeding point, he or she will then usually ligate it if it is small, and suture-ligate it if it is large. From an assistant's viewpoint, the task is similar: you must make it easier for the surgeon to place the ligature material around the clip, and then remove the clip at the correct time.

### Removing ligature clips

When removing clips with your right hand, simply use a similar grip as recommended for using scissors (see Figure 10.2). However, unlike when using the scissors, it is not necessary to stabilise the instrument with the left hand. This is because the clip is already anchored by its point of attachment at the tips.

Like normal household scissors, most surgical instruments are designed for use by right-handed people. This includes artery clips. Therefore, placing and removing these instruments with the right hand is easy, but most people find that doing so with the left hand is difficult. However, this is because most people, when called upon to use their left hand to release a clip, naturally use a left-handed grip that is simply a mirror image of their normal right-handed grip. Because of the way the instruments are sprung, this is awkward and clumsy. This is an important point, because it commonly occurs that as an assistant, you are required to remove a clip with your left hand because your right hand is occupied elsewhere. To overcome this problem, use the left-handed grip shown in Figure 10.21. Push down with your thumb while giving counter-pressure upwards with your middle finger. This grip can also be used for scissors, although for some reason, it seems to be less commonly required for them.

A third clip-releasing technique exists, which might be called a 'reverse right-handed' grip (see Figure 10.22). It is occasionally useful when the clip is lying rather horizontally, with the tips pointing towards your body. In this situation, the normal right-handed grip can be awkward because it requires excessive

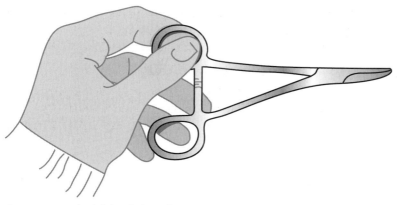

**Figure 10.21**   The left-handed grip for releasing clips. The middle and ring ringer exert counter-pressure against the thumb and index finger.

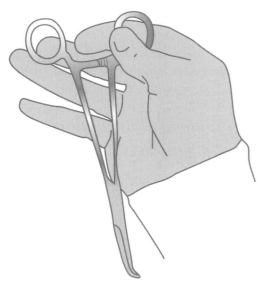

**Figure 10.22**   The 'reverse right-handed' grip for releasing clips. This is similar to the left-handed grip, in that the middle and ring fingers give counter-pressure against the thumb and index finger, to release the clip ratchet.

pronation at the wrist. As with the left-hand grip, push down with your thumb against counter-pressure from your middle finger.

These grips are not difficult to master. They can easily be practised at home, simply using normal household scissors to cut scrap paper. Although such scissors will not have a ratchet mechanism, this does not matter much, because the basic elements of the grip itself and the finger pressures required still apply.

Although the left-handed grip (and to a lesser extent, the reverse right-handed grip) described above are important to master, they do not give quite the same degree of fine control as the normal right-handed grip. Therefore, it is probably better to use the normal right-handed grip whenever practical, rather than using another grip simply for the sake of being clever.

The act of removing the clip is a three-step process (see Figure 10.23):

1 When the surgeon indicates that he or she is about to ligate a clipped vessel, grasp the clip's handles gently, and raise them (Figure 10.23(a)). This makes it easier for the surgeon to pass the tie under the handles.

2 The surgeon will now pass the ligature around the instrument tips. Lowering the handles slightly at this point will make this easier, by raising the tips away from the adjacent tissue (Figure 10.23(b)). (*Note*: Sometimes the surgeon may pass the ligature under the tips before the handles.)

3 The surgeon will make the first throw of a surgical knot (usually a reef knot). Release the clip carefully as the surgeon tightens this throw around the vessel; the surgeon will often ask for the clip to be removed at the correct time. This request may be the single word 'Off'. Timing is important. The aim is for you to remove the clip at the same moment that the surgeon tightens the ligature around the vessel. If you remove the clip too soon (before the ligature has

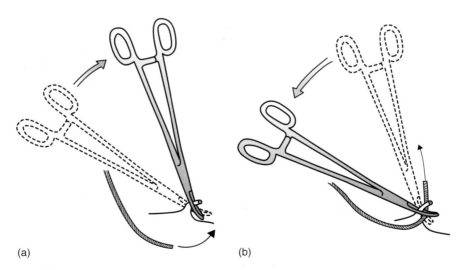

(a)                                                      (b)

**Figure 10.23**   Raising and lowering clips to allow the surgeon to pass a ligature around a clipped vessel. (a) First, raise the clip handles gently to allow the surgeon to pass the ligature underneath the handles. (b) Then carefully lower the handles using the vessel as a fulcrum. This raises the instrument tips, allowing the surgeon to pass the ligature under them, and therefore around the vessel.

taken hold of the vessel), the vessel is likely to spring away and not be captured by the ligature. If you release too late (after the knot has been tightened), the ligature will be loose on the vessel, and may slip off it later.

During the entire procedure, you must handle the clip very gently to avoid tearing the vessel. However, once the clip is safely clear of the vessel and ligature, you can remove your hand quickly, pass the clip off to the scrub nurse, and get ready for the next step (usually cutting the ligature). To help you handle the clip gently when performing manoeuvres 1 and 2 above, you may find it helpful to imagine that the point where the clip grasps the vessel is like the fulcrum of a children's see-saw. That is, when you raise the handles and then the tips, the fulcrum should remain stationary.

Gentleness is also enhanced by cradling the clip loosely during this manoeuvre, rather than grasping it firmly.

### Loaded ties

When a vessel in an awkward place needs to be ligated (typically, at the bottom of a deep surgical wound), it is often not possible to place a ligature around the clip with the unaided hands. In this case, the ligature may be mounted in a pair of long forceps (e.g. De Bakey's) and passed down into the wound.

A more common and perhaps less awkward method is to mount the ligature at the end of a second long angled clip, such as a Lahey. From here it is passed around the vessel, near the tips of the first clip deep in the wound. This clip with a length of suture material mounted in its jaws is known as a 'loaded tie'. If the suture material in a loaded tie is not mounted correctly, it may be difficult to place it where it is needed. The suture material should be mounted at the tip of the clip, forming a bowstring. If it is mounted away from the tips, it can be difficult to manoeuvre effectively (see Figure 10.24).

The 'loaded tie' technique is also used when slinging a tape around a major tubular structure (e.g. the bile duct or the femoral artery). The purpose of this tape may be to act as a gentle retractor, or in the case of major blood vessels, it may be used as a method of controlling blood loss. In this slinging technique, the surgeon dissects a plane around the structure, and places an angled clip through this plane. The surgeon then opens the jaws of this clip to receive the loaded tape, which will usually be handled by you, the assistant (see also 'vascular surgery', p. 173).

In a variation of this slinging technique, a slightly different method of mounting the loaded tie is used. In the method described above, it is usually the 'bowstring' part of the tie that you insert into the waiting jaws of the surgeon's instrument (Figure 10.24, middle). An alternative is to insert the small part that projects beyond the tips of your clip (Figure 10.24, top).

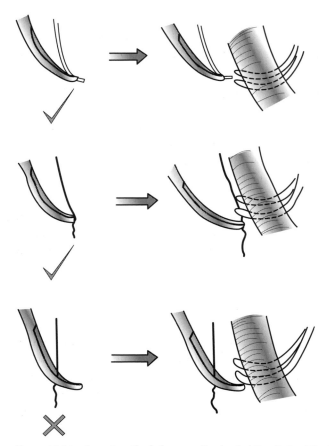

**Figure 10.24** Correct methods for mounting loaded ties. Both of the top two methods are correct. Note how, in the bottom figure, the tie is too far away from the tips of the instrument. This creates difficulty when attempting to pass the ligature into the jaws of the surgeon's clip.

Both methods are satisfactory, with slightly different advantages and disadvantages. The second method described above, is useful where there is limited space to place your clip underneath the surgeon's, and stiff material such as a rubber 'loop' is being inserted. This method also enables the tip of the 'loop' to be inserted in to the waiting jaws, which means that as the jaws are then withdrawn, less trauma is inflicted on the tissues.

However, if the distal piece of ligature is soft and floppy, its floppiness can make it difficult to manoeuvre into the narrow space between the jaws of the surgeon's clip. In this event, the 'bowstring' method probably gives slightly better overall control.

## Clip and double-tie

This is really just a variant of the simple clip-and-tie manoeuvre (see above) with the obvious exception that the vessel is ligated twice. It is sometimes used on larger vessels, for extra security.

There are several different ways of achieving the second tie. Sometimes two clamps are used, in which case each ligating manoeuvre is identical to the clip-and-tie method. Generally, the clamp that is further from the cut end of the vessel is removed first. To remove the other clamp first would mean having to manoeuvre the tie between the clips, which is awkward.

A second method of double-ligating a vessel uses just one clamp. This method is known as the 'ease and squeeze' method. As the name suggests, as the clamp is released, the surgeon tightens the knot as usual, but instead of the assistant removing the clamp, the clamp is closed again on the vessel. A second ligature is then applied to the vessel. When assisting at this method, it is important that in the initial release of the clamp (the 'ease'), the jaws are eased open only far enough to allow the ligature to tighten on the vessel.

## Suture

The surgeon usually sutures bleeding points without any special assistance needed, other than to keep the field clear of blood. The commonest method for small to moderate-sized bleeding points is the figure-of-eight stitch. The name describes the configuration in which the suture material lies after it has been placed and tied, although since part of it is buried in the tissues, it looks more like the figure 'X' than the figure '8'.

## Transfixion-ligation

This technique is used for larger vessels. Essentially, it is a form of ligation, with the variation that a needle is used to pass the suture material through the vessel (i.e. it transfixes the vessel). This greatly reduces the possibility of the suture material slipping off the vessel.

## Tying ligatures

As noted previously (p. 5), in some operations, it can be difficult to distinguish the surgeon from the assistant. There are several intra-operative tasks which assistants may occasionally be asked to perform, but which are better described as surgical skills than assistant skills. These tasks include tying ligatures, and sometimes wound closure, especially skin suturing. They are well described in other textbooks, and the reader is referred to some of these in the section 'Suggested further reading', p. 201.

## Preventing suture material from tangling

### 'Following' a suture line (see also p. 61 and p.178)

When a surgeon is tying interrupted sutures, your role as an assistant will usually be simply to cut the sutures (see p. 57). However, if the surgeon is performing a continuous suture, you may be asked to hold the suture material steady. This is known as 'following' the suture. There are two reasons for doing this. The first reason is simply to hold the suture material out of the surgeon's way, while the second is to maintain the tension on the suture that has already been placed, so that it does not become loose. This second reason may be compared to threading a bootlace on a long boot. If the first few throws of the lace are not kept tight, they will quickly work loose, and are more difficult to tighten once the whole boot has been laced.

However, unlike lacing a boot, it is very important not to over-tighten sutures in a wound. Doing so can strangulate the tissues contained within the suture, so that they become ischaemic and die. In almost all surgery, the goal of surgical sutures is to hold tissues gently together so that the body can heal the wound. This is summarised in the surgical maxim 'Appose, don't necrose'. Importantly, most surgeons will hand you the suture at the angle and tension that they want you to maintain. Grasp the suture material firmly, and continue holding it at that angle and tension, until the surgeon has placed the next stitch. The proper moment to release your grasp is just after that next stitch has been placed, and the surgeon is pulling it taught to the correct tension. It takes some practice to release the suture at exactly the right moment. If you release too soon, the suture will flop loosely and the correct tension on the wound edges may be lost. If you release too late, the surgeon will be tugging the suture from your grasp, which some surgeons find annoying.

When 'following' sutures, the correct place to grasp the suture material is usually so that you take one-third of the free suture material, and leave two-thirds for the surgeon (see Figure 10.25). If you grasp too close to the needle, the surgeon will not have enough material to work with. Conversely, if you grasp too close to the wound, the excess suture material will flop around and get in the surgeon's way. This 'one-third:two-thirds' rule may need to be ignored when the suture material is very short or very long. When the suture is very short, you will need to give the surgeon more to work with (or perhaps let go altogether), and when it is very long, you may need to take more to prevent it getting in the way.

Some suture materials, especially monofilaments, are difficult to grip with surgical gloves, as they become very slippery. You may find that they will slip from your grasp if you simply hold them between fingers and thumb. Therefore, when

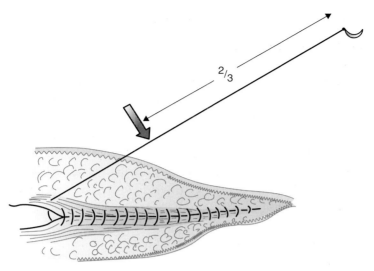

**Figure 10.25** 'Following' a suture. Showing the correct site to grasp the suture; take one-third of the free suture, giving two-thirds to the surgeon.

'following' sutures, learn to grip suture material with an interlocking grip (such as that shown in Figure 10.26), which prevents this from occurring.

## Placing packs to protect suture material

Suture material has an extraordinary ability to entangle itself in surrounding objects. In particular, it often snags on instruments in or near the surgical wound, such as artery clips and retractors. Self-retaining retractors are an especially common site of snagging. To help minimise the problem, it is sometimes appropriate simply to drape a sterile pack over the snagging object. Some surgeons prefer these packs to be moistened beforehand. This is because dry packs may have a drying, and therefore theoretically injurious, effect on exposed tissues. More practically, a moist pack is heavier, and so less likely to be dislodged, and perhaps allows suture material to slide over it more easily.

## Drains

Many different designs of drain exist. Broadly, they are simple devices used to evacuate fluid from the body. Some drains (especially chest drains) also drain gas. A typical drain is a piece of hollow plastic tubing placed in a surgical wound at the end of the operation. Its purpose is to drain fluid or gas that would otherwise accumulate in the wound. Some types have a sharp spike on one end, which

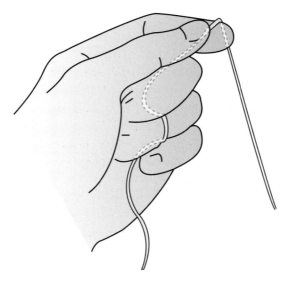

**Figure 10.26**  Non-slip grip for 'following' sutures. This is particularly useful for monofilaments used to close long wounds (e.g. laparotomy wounds).

is used to drive the drain through the tissues from the depths of the wound to the exterior. The spike is usually cut off the drain as soon as it has completed this task.

Surgeons will usually place drains themselves. As an assistant, your role will typically be to cut off the spike, to cut the drain to the correct length, and to trim the suture holding it in place. Unless directed otherwise, cut the spike off close to its join with the drain tubing, to give the surgeon the maximum length of tubing. When the drain is being cut to length, often the surgeon will hold it up in a way that exposes an approximately 5 cm length of it, between his or her hands. He or she will then invite you to cut the drain at that exposed length. Few things are as tough on scissors as cutting a surgical drain, so always ask the scrub nurse for the correct scissors. Usually, they will be a sturdy pair of Ferguson or Mayo type (see Figure 10.1), but in your request, it is best simply to refer to them as as 'a pair of scissors to cut the drain, please.' Once the drain has been placed, it is usually sutured in place, to prevent later dislodgement. It is often helpful if you hold the drain up vertically away from the patient's body, while the surgeon ties the suture around the drain.

## Prosthetic materials

Many different types of operations use prosthetic materials. The commoner prostheses include artificial intra-ocular lenses, plastic mesh used for hernia repairs, plastic grafts in arterial surgery, and artificial hip-joints and heart valves made of metal alloys and plastic.

Like any artificial material introduced into the tissues, a prosthesis is a foreign body, albeit a beneficial one. An important point common to all foreign bodies, is that infection of them is difficult to treat. Antibiotics seldom eradicate established infection of a foreign body, and treatment is often unsuccessful without removal of the foreign body. Hence, prosthetic infection is a dreaded complication of any surgery where prosthetic material is implanted. The need for removal of an infected prosthesis is usually something of a disaster, not only because (at least in theory), it is a preventable re-do operation, but also because it leaves behind an infected surgical 'bed'. Any replacement prosthesis placed in this 'bed' is also likely to become infected.

Therefore, when implanting prosthetic materials, most surgeons will insist on meticulous adherence to sterile conditions. Any breach of these conditions is likely to trigger unhappiness in the surgeon. If you are the source of the breach, most surgeons will promptly delegate the task of feeling unhappy, to you. However, the surgeon's wrath will be greater if you fail to notice your error, and far greater still if he or she suspects that you did notice it, but have attempted to conceal it. In the eyes of most surgeons, the first two of the above errors are forgivable, but the third is not.

As an assistant, you are therefore strongly advised to share the surgeon's concern for sterility. In particular, avoid touching prosthetic materials unless the surgeon asks you to do so. This is because surgical gloves commonly harbour small numbers of bacteria, which are normally unimportant, but are enough to cause infection of a prosthesis. If you must handle prosthetic material, try to do so with sterile instruments such as a pair of forceps or a clip, rather than your gloved hands. If you do make a mistake that causes a breach in the sterile field, apologetically notify the surgeon immediately.

# Assisting at special types of surgery

# Part III

# Cardiothoracic surgery

## 11

**Craig Jurisevic** MBBS MS FRACS

Cardiothoracic Unit, Royal Adelaide Hospital, Adelaide, South Australia

## ■ Introduction

The principles of assisting at cardiac and thoracic surgical operations are no different from those of other specialties. Maintenance of a stable, bloodless and well exposed operative field is the primary goal. This is much more easily achieved in cardiac than in thoracic surgical procedures, thanks to the aid of a cardiopulmonary bypass pump, minimal blood in the field, and a still heart. By contrast, in thoracic surgical procedures the assistant and surgeon must contend with mobile lung tissue, a beating heart and a continuously shifting mediastinum due to ventilation on the non-operated lung. As with other surgical specialties, your role as the assistant is crucial in maintaining the ideal environment for the surgeon to complete his or her procedure effectively.

It is important that the patient's investigations are available pre-operatively for the surgeon to review. In particular, if a coronary artery bypass is to be performed, the patient's angiogram results (and preferably, the films themselves) should be available. In thoracic surgery, the patient's chest X-rays and/or thoracic CT scans should be available.

## Assisting at cardiac surgery
### ■ The median sternotomy

The median sternotomy is by far the commonest incision for heart operations. It involves making a vertical skin incision from just below the sternal notch down to the xiphisternum. Once the skin is incised, only subcutaneous fat remains to be divided before the periosteum of the sternum is reached. The surgeon will score the sternal periosteum from the top of the manubrium down to the xiphisternum and will divide the xiphisternum. During this stage, you should retract the skin and fat of both sides of the sternotomy wound.

Next, the surgeon will cut the sternum vertically, using a saw that looks very similar to a hand-held domestic 'jig-saw', starting from below (the xiphisternal end). This is known as 'splitting the sternum'. You will be required to use a Kocher retractor to retract the skin at the top end of the incision, and protect it from the saw. You should also hold a Yankauer sucker to keep the field clean while the surgeon saws from below upwards. This can be quite a bloody procedure, as the periosteum and medulla of the sternum are very vascular. Once the sternum has been 'split', the surgeon will place a pack between the split ends underneath the sternum. You will be required to retract the skin edges and use the sucker, whilst the surgeon diathermies the periosteal edges of the anterior and posterior table of the sternum.

The surgeon will then place a self-retaining retractor (almost always a Finochietto type) and retract the sternal edges open. This displays the thymic fat and the pericardium. The surgeon will now dissect the thymic fat. To assist with this step, you should use a pair of De Bakey forceps to provide counter-traction (see p. 51–3), following the surgeon from the top of the wound to inferiorly. You will then be asked to grasp the pericardium with the De Bakey's forceps, whilst the surgeon perforates it, this being followed by diathermy of the anterior aspect of the pericardium in a linear fashion to expose the heart.

The next step is to place retraction sutures bilaterally in the pericardium, to expose the heart and lift the heart anteriorly. These retraction sutures are commonly placed around each side of the Finochietto retractor and tied in place. However, if the surgeon is going to harvest the mammary artery (see below), these pericardial sutures will be placed after that step.

## ■ Harvesting the internal mammary artery

For most coronary artery bypass grafting procedures, the left internal thoracic artery (often known by its former name of internal mammary artery) is harvested. This provides an arterial graft with its origin left undisturbed.

A special sternal retractor will be used to elevate the left side of the sternum, leaving the under surface of the left chest wall exposed, ready for the surgeon to harvest the mammary artery pedicle. At this stage, your role will usually be simply to suction away the diathermy smoke. Once the internal mammary artery is harvested, then the surgeon will remove the mammary retractor and replace it with a Finochietto retractor. At this stage the pericardium will be opened and the pericardial stay sutures will be placed. The heart can then be cannulated for cardiopulmonary bypass.

# ■ Cannulation of the heart for cardiopulmonary bypass

This procedure involves the placement of a large-bore venous cannula into the right atrial appendage, or, where a bi-caval system is used, also into the inferior vena cava through a separate incision in the right atrium. This venous cannula takes blood to the perfusion pump, where it is oxygenated before returning to the body via a cannula inserted in the aortic root.

During this part of the operation, you will be required to hold the venous and arterial cannulae once the surgeon has inserted them in their respective sites. The surgeon will insert stay sutures around the base of each cannula, while you hold the cannula and the stay sutures in place. At this point cardiopulmonary bypass is commenced.

The aortic cannula will be placed in the ascending aorta, and secured in place with reinforced purse-string sutures. Cardiopulmonary bypass is then instituted.

You will notice that the heart will empty, ready for the surgeon to insert another aortic root cannula through which a cardioplegic (cardiac arresting) fluid can be inserted. Again, the surgeon will ask you to hold the cardioplegic cannula in the aortic root, whilst he or she fixes it in position. The surgeon will next apply a cross-clamp above the cardioplegic cannula but below the aortic cannula, and then ask for the perfusionist (bypass pump technician) to start infusing the cardioplegia. Within 30 s or so the heart will arrest, and the surgeon will have an essentially still and bloodless field.

# ■ Harvesting of the long saphenous vein and radial artery for grafting

Depending on the particular conduit required by the surgeon, either the long saphenous vein, the radial artery in the forearm, or both will be harvested. Assisting in either of these procedures is quite simple and involves retracting the skin flap on either side of the long saphenous vein or radial artery, whilst the surgeon mobilises the vessel. There will be ligation of side branches and you will be required to cut the proximal side branch sutures once the surgeon has mobilised the branches. For further tips on assisting at the harvest of vein grafts (see 'vascular surgery', p. 175).

# ■ Coronary bypass grafting

Once the heart has arrested and the conduits are prepared, the surgeon will commence grafting. To start, the surgeon will make a small arteriotomy in the coronary artery, at the site where the bypass graft is to be placed. This will often be bloodless, but because of collateral blood flow, some blood may ooze from the arteriotomy site. To combat this, you will be provided with a 20 mL syringe with a pipette attached, filled with heparinised saline. Gently squirt away any blood, whilst the surgeon is anastomosing the graft to the coronary artery. It is not uncommon for a junior assistant, in the heat of the moment, to spray madly on the surface of the heart, showering the surgeon and other staff with a film of normal saline. This should be avoided; the objective is to provide just enough gentle irrigation to provide the surgeon with a bloodless field, without significant trauma to the coronary artery or the bypass graft.

As well as providing the surgeon with a bloodless field, you will often be asked to follow the suture with your left hand, whilst the surgeon is performing the anastomosis (see also p. 88 and 178). Commonly, fine sutures, such as 5/0 or 6/0 Prolene will be used, and these require very little tension. Excessive tension will result in the suture tearing through the coronary artery, the graft, or both, or it may result in breakage of the suture. This is often felt to be the most difficult part of the procedure for the assistant. It is however, the most crucial part of the operation, and a delicate hand is appreciated.

Once the distal ends of the anastomosis are completed, the surgeon will then anastomose the proximal ends (if the graft is a saphenous vein or radial artery) to the aortic root. Again, you will be required to follow the advancing suture and occasionally squirt blood out of the aortic root with the syringe of heparinised saline. When the surgeon finishes each anastomosis, he or she will have to tie the suture. You can help by squirting a small amount of saline on the surgeon's thumb and index finger to prevent any snagging, whilst tying down the knot (for further tips on this technique, see also 'vascular surgery', p. 178).

## ■ Coming off cardiopulmonary bypass

Once the grafts have been found to be functioning adequately, the surgeon will plan to discontinue cardiopulmonary bypass. This is a very standardised process. The surgeon will ask the perfusionist to reduce the drainage from the heart, thus gradually allowing the heart to take over from the bypass machine. Once the heart is off bypass, the surgeon will then remove the venous cannula. To prevent atmospheric air entering the heart, this procedure requires simultaneous removal of the cannula and snugging down of the purse-string suture at the right atrial appendage (and the right atrium in the region of the inferior vena cava if a double-venous cannula system is used). Usually, the surgeon will remove the venous cannula while you snug down the purse-string. Snug it down at the exact moment the surgeon removes the cannula. Next, the surgeon will ask you to hold the purse-string suture up, while he or she places a further reinforcing suture around its base. The final step after weaning from bypass is removal of the aortic cannula and the surgeon will, again, ask you to snug down the purse-string suture as the aortic cannula is removed. The surgeon will again place a reinforcing suture over the aortic cannulation site.

## ■ Insertion of drains after a median sternotomy

The surgeon will place, one, two or three drains within the mediastinum, left and/or right pleura depending on whether or not the pleural had been opened. These are usually placed through the skin in the upper aspect of the epigastrium and are fixed with silk sutures. As when a surgeon is placing any other drain in the body, you can assist by holding the drain up (see p. 89).

## ■ Closure of the sternotomy

This is done by placing five to eight interrupted sutures through both sides of the sternum. Importantly, the suture material is stainless-steel wire, which is handled differently to other suture materials, so your role as assistant is also different. Unlike most other suture material which is secured in place by knotting it, a wire suture is secured by simply twisting its two ends tightly together. The sternal wires are twisted and reinforced at the anterior aspect of the sternotomy.

To allow the best access, the sternal edges are not brought together, and the wires are not tied (or rather, twisted), until all of them have been placed. That is, each time a wire is placed through the sternum, the needle is cut off and then an artery clip is placed on each free end. Once all the wire sutures are in place, you will be asked to hold up each wire suture sequentially, prior to the surgeon twisting each one in turn. After this you will be asked to hold all the wires and their attached artery clips together, so that the surgeon can cut the wires. The surgeon will then close the fascia, fat and skin.

## ■ Assisting in aortic valve, mitral valve or tricuspid valve surgery

The same principles mentioned in the previous sections apply. An additional feature is that you will be responsible for keeping the aortic root or mitral annulus free of debris (using the Yankauer sucker) during the resection of the aortic and mitral valve, respectively. This is a very important task, as any debris that you fail to remove can later embolise, with potentially catastrophic consequences.

Multiple interrupted sutures are used to secure cardiac valves in place. Usually, the 'parachute' technique is used for implanting cardiac valves (see p. 177 and 61, and Figure 10.7). That is, each suture is placed in the valve and its bed, and then the two free ends of the suture material are clipped together for later tying. You can help to prevent these clips entangling by threading the finger-rings sequentially along another instrument, such as a Roberts clamp (see Figure 109–17).

# Assisting at thoracic surgery

## ■ Introduction

As in many other types of surgery, thoracic surgery can broadly be categorised into 'open' surgery (usually thoracotomy) and endoscopic ('thoracoscopic') surgery. Assisting at open thoracic surgery tends to be more physically demanding than in cardiac surgical procedures or thoracoscopy. You may be required to retract strongly for several minutes, or occasionally hours (see below).

In open thoracotomy procedures, exposure can be extremely variable depending on the patient's size, chest wall shape and intra-thoracic pathology. Your main role when assisting at any thoracic surgical procedure is to provide the surgeon with adequate exposure in what can be a difficult operative field.

## ■ Video-assisted thoracoscopic procedures

Video-assisted thoracoscopic procedures (also known as video-assisted thoracotomy, or more commonly, VAT) are performed using techniques similar to those in laparoscopic surgery. However, a major difference between thoracoscopic and laparoscopic surgery is that in laparoscopic surgery, the abdominal wall's elasticity means that gas must be insufflated into the abdomen to create a space in which to operate. In contrast, gas insufflation is not needed in VAT. This is because the ribs make the thorax comparatively rigid, so that once a port site is made and the pleural space opened, the lung simply falls away from the chest wall (providing there are no significant pleural adhesions). The opposite lung remains inflated, allowing ventilation; this is possible because, in thoracoscopic surgery, the anaesthetist uses a double-lumen endotracheal tube, which allows for isolated ventilation of individual lungs.

In all thoracoscopic procedures you, the assistant, will hold the thoracoscope. In some procedures you may also be required to retract the lung via a thoracoscopic retractor. However, this is uncommon because the lung can usually be pushed out of the way, giving adequate exposure without the need for a retraction device.

Compared with most cardiac surgical procedures and most open thoracotomy procedures, you will find that your role in tissue manipulation is quite limited. However, your role in driving the camera is crucial. Most of the points of technique that apply to laparoscopic assisting, apply equally to assisting at VAT procedures. It is therefore suggested that you also refer to the chapter on assisting at laparoscopic surgery, especially pp. 109–17 (camera technique). In particular, you should keep the point of dissection in the centre of the camera field at all times.

# ■ Open thoracic surgery

## Specific situations in thoracic surgery

### Thoracotomy and major lung resections

A pneumonectomy is a resection of an entire lung, while a lobectomy is the resection of a lobe of the lung. For some lung cancer resections the patient may require a bi-lobectomy where adjacent lobes are resected, or a smaller resection known as a segmentectomy. A segmentectomy is an anatomical dissection of a pulmonary segment to include the segmental pulmonary artery, pulmonary vein and bronchus. From the assistant's point of view there is very little difference between any of these operations. However, if the surgeon plans to perform a pneumonectomy from the outset, this is often much faster than performing a lobectomy, as the lobar or segmental blood vessels and airways need not be dissected.

All these major lung resections are performed through a thoracotomy. The commonest types of thoracotomy are the postero-lateral thoracotomy, and the limited thoracotomy (occasionally known as the mini-thoracotomy). For all of these operations, your role involves sequentially retracting each soft tissue layer (skin, fat and muscle), as it is divided. Once the intercostal space (usually the fifth) is reached, the surgeon will ask you to retract the scapula with a scapula retractor. This is quite a difficult and physically demanding manoeuvre. Retract the scapula superiorly along the chest wall rather than trying to lift it up in the air. You will usually be required to do this until the pleural space is entered, at which point the surgeon will place a self-retaining intercostal retractor into the intercostal space. This is the most physically demanding part of the thoracotomy for you, as you may be required to hold the scapula firmly in position for up to 5–8 min.

As the operation proceeds, you will be required to retract the lung in various positions. The most commonly used instrument for retracting lung tissue is a 'swab-on-a-stick' (see p. 82). Another device called a lung retractor or lung whisk, (which looks vaguely similar to a simple kitchen whisk) can be used to retract a lobe, or the entire lung. During dissection of the mediastinum and the hilum, you will also be required to use a Yankauer sucker to keep the operative field relatively blood free.

Once the resection is completed, you will need to retract the scapula again while the surgeon places a series of peri-costal interrupted sutures to approximate the ribs. After the remaining lung has been re-inflated, the rib approximation sutures are tied and you can release the scapular retractor.

## Correction of chest wall deformities

Repair of pectus excavatum (hollow chest) or pectus carinatum (pigeon chest) deformity is a physically demanding procedure for the surgeon and for you, the assistant. This is because, typically, it takes between 2 and 3 h and you will be required to retract strongly for most of that time. Briefly, it entails the surgeon raising large extramuscular flaps (which you retract) and then sequentially resecting part of the third to eighth costal cartilages bilaterally. These resections are done via muscle-splitting incisions, while you retract the edges.

# Laparoscopic surgery

12

**Comus Whalan** BMBS MD FRACS

Noarlunga Health Service, Adelaide, South Australia

## ■ Introduction

Laparoscopic surgery is a method of performing intra-abdominal operations through small incisions (typically less than 2 cm). It has developed at a rapid rate since the late 1980s. At least initially, this was largely because of technological advances that allowed good-quality video cameras to be made small enough to be held easily in the hand.

Using a miniaturised video camera and specialised instruments inserted through these small incisions, the surgeon can now do operations that previously needed much larger incisions. The advantages of this are not merely cosmetic; usually, the patient's recovery is quicker, and sometimes dramatically so. For example, after laparoscopic cholecystectomy, patients typically stay in hospital for less than 24 h, whereas after open cholecystectomy, a stay of almost a week is usual.

The same technological advances that have allowed laparoscopic surgery to develop, have also allowed minimal-access surgery to develop in other areas, such as thoracic surgery and surgery of the paranasal sinuses.

## ■ Setting up for laparoscopic operations

### General layout of instruments

There is a lot of individual variation in the way surgeons arrange their instruments for most operations, and this particularly applies to laparoscopic operations. However, the general principles are described below.

There are six lines (i.e. cords, cables and tubes) that have one end on the operating table, and the other end attached to an unsterile object nearby. The six lines are the light cord, the camera and diathermy cables, and tubing for the gas, irrigation and suction. A mnemonic for these cords is 'Lights, Camera, Suction! Gas–Fire–Water.'

When setting up for an operation, all these lines are initially on the scrub nurse's tray of sterile instruments, so they are initially sterile along their entire length. Obviously, however, one end must be handed off the operating table to a non-scrubbed member of the surgical team, to connect to its appropriate apparatus. On some of these cords, the two ends look quite similar, but are subtly different. One end is designed to attach only to the 'on-table' equipment, and the other only to the 'off-table' equipment. Make sure you do not hand off the wrong end. This mistake is particularly easy to make with the light cable.

Some of the 'off-table' equipment, to which the above cords are attached (including the $CO_2$ cylinder and insufflator, light source and camera unit) is arranged as a 'stack' or 'tower' on a special trolley.

Most surgeons will ensure all the laparoscopic equipment is properly arranged, and ready for immediate use, before making any incisions.

## Camera and associated instruments

The laparoscopic camera (see Figures 12.1 and 12.2).

The camera head is about the size of two matchboxes together. It is designed to be held in the hand, and this usually means the assistant's hand. One end has a locking ring, into which the laparoscope is inserted. The other end has a cable protruding from it. This cable is plugged into the camera box on the laparoscopic tower.

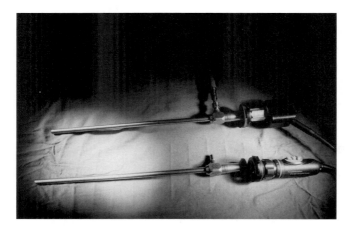

**Figure 12.1** Laparoscopic equipment. Top: a 0° laparoscope has been assembled with light cord and camera attached. Bottom: the light cord and camera have not yet been attached to a 30° laparoscope. Note the different angulation of the tips of the 0° and 30° scopes.

## The light cord

This is a flexible fibre-optic cable, slightly thicker than an average ballpoint pen. It is made of numerous very fine glass fibres that transmit light. Bending it excessively breaks these fibres, decreasing the amount of light transmitted. If a light cord seems dim, you can test for broken fibres with the so-called 'salt and pepper test'.

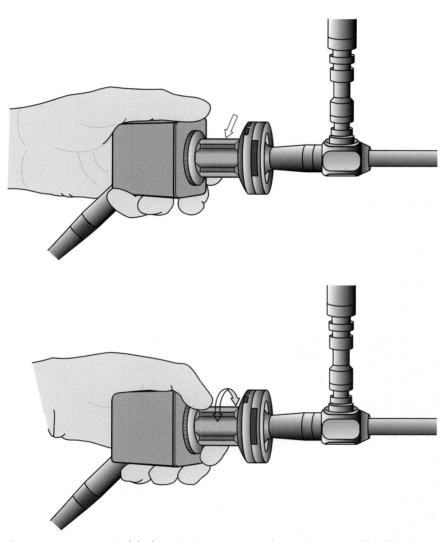

**Figure 12.2**  Correct grip of the laparoscopic camera. Top: the camera rests comfortably in the hand, with the index finger and thumb close to, but not touching, the focussing ring (arrowed). Bottom: this grip allows the index finger and thumb to reach forward easily and adjust the focus.

Hold one end of the cord up to a bright light, such as the operating theatre lights. Look at the other end of the cord. You will see a bright circle of light, but with a number of tiny black specks on it ('the pepper in the salt'). These black specks are broken glass fibres, which do not transmit the light. Even new cords may have a few broken fibres, but you will soon develop a sense of what is an excessive number. This test can also be used on other instruments that contain glass fibres, such as laparoscopes themselves. Do not use the laparoscopic light source itself as your light for the 'salt and pepper test'. The light is far too bright and will simply dazzle you.

### The laparoscope (see Figure12.1)

This is a rod-shaped instrument, typically about 1 cm in diameter, and 40 cm long. One end has an eye-piece similar to those on binoculars. This end is attached to the laparoscopic camera. The other end is inserted into the peritoneal cavity via a port (see below). The most common variety of laparoscope 'looks straight ahead' out the end (like a normal telescope), and is known as a 0° scope (pronounced zero-degree or nought-degree). Other scopes, known as angled scopes, look out at an angle to the end, like a periscope. Various degrees of angulation (e.g. 30°) are available. Angled scopes are easy to identify, because the degree of angulation is inscribed on the shaft of the scope, and the tip of the scope is visibly angulated.

Once the laparoscope or light cable are connected to the light source, avoid pointing them at people's faces, including your own. The light is very bright and causes uncomfortable dazzling. It is also bad practice to allow the tip to remain in contact with the surgical drapes, as with some types there is a theoretical risk of burning the drapes, or worse still, the patient.

### Gas

$CO_2$ gas is released at a controlled rate from a cylinder, by a machine known as an insufflator. It is conveyed by a plastic tube from the insufflator to one of the ports; usually the port that is used for the laparoscope.

### White balance

When the camera is first set up at the start of a laparoscopic operation, the camera must be programmed to reproduce different colours accurately. This is known as the 'white balance' or 'white set'. It is quite simple to do. The tip of the laparoscope is merely held a few centimetres away from a white object (usually a sterile pack), and the white balance button is pressed. In some models, the button is on the camera itself. In others, it is on the camera box on the laparoscopic tower, and so obviously must be pressed by a non-scrubbed member of the surgical team. Once the button is pressed, the white balance process takes about three seconds. Most units inform you when the process is complete, either by flashing words to that effect on the screen, or by emitting a characteristic beep.

When performing a white balance, it is important that the white object occupies the entire visual field of the camera, for the whole of the few seconds after the button is pressed. If the camera strays even partly on to an object of some other colour, the white balance will be incorrect, and colours on the screen will be abnormal.

## Ports

Essentially, these are tubes placed in the abdominal wall so that they form a tunnel between the peritoneal cavity and the outside. They have valves that allow instruments to pass into the peritoneal cavity, while limiting loss of the insufflated $CO_2$ gas. They are made in a variety of different diameters, with the most common ranging from 5 to 12 mm. There is even a type large enough to allow the surgeon's hand to enter the peritoneal cavity (for so-called hand-assisted laparoscopic surgery), although this type is not in common use.

Ports must be inserted carefully to avoid injury to underlying abdominal organs. This is especially so for the first port, which is almost always the port through which the laparoscope itself will be inserted.

The method of inserting the first port is different to that of the subsequent ports. Several different techniques exist, and like so many things in surgery, each surgeon seems to have his or her own minor variations on the technique. The commonest is probably the direct vision technique, also known as the open cut-down method. In this method, the surgeon makes an initial skin incision (usually at the umbilicus) and then dissects down to the peritoneum. A hole is made in the peritoneum, and the port is inserted either with a blunt trochar, or by threading it over a blunt plastic rod.

There are many different variations on the open cut-down technique. However, many surgeons like the assistant to use a Rutherford–Morison (also known as a Littlewood) retractor to grasp the skin of the umbilicus, and pull it upwards. A second such instrument is then often placed on the umbilical stalk (cicatrix), and again, pulled upwards by the assistant. The surgeon will then incise the peritoneum. It is important to pull upwards (i.e. towards the ceiling) during this procedure, because this allows the underlying bowel to fall away from the wound as the peritoneum is incised, and air enters the cavity. Pulling upwards also makes the depths of the wound easier to see. For the same reason, many surgeons ask the assistant to use a small Langenbeck's retractor to retract the skin, exposing the umbilical stalk.

A variant of this technique involves attaching the camera to specially designed ports, such as the 'Visiport™' (Autosuture) or 'Optiview™' (Ethicon Endo-Surgery). These ports have a transparent cutting blade at the advancing edge, placed in such a way that the surgeon can watch as the port cuts through the tissues into the peritoneum.

Another common method for establishing pneumoperitoneum is the Veres needle technique. The Veres needle is a special spring-loaded needle that is inserted carefully through the abdominal wall. Gas is then insufflated through the needle, and the first port inserted blindly with a sharp trochar.

Once the first port has been inserted, the laparoscope is inserted through it and used to watch the subsequent ports entering the peritoneal cavity, so insertion of these ports is usually easier. Subsequent ports are often referred to as 'working ports', because they convey the operating instruments. They are usually inserted by pushing them through the abdominal wall with a sharp trochar, while watching entry of the trochar on the monitor screen (see p. 110 and Figure 12.4).

## Instruments

These may loosely be categorised into instruments that are stored in the quiver, and instruments that are kept on the scrub nurse's trolley.

## Quiver instruments

### Sucker-irrigator

This is an instrument operated by the surgeon. There are many different designs, some of which include the diathermy instrument (see below). Typically, it is a modified tube about 40 cm long, usually with a handle containing two valve buttons resembling those found on a trumpet. One button causes irrigation fluid (usually normal saline) to flow from the end. The other button activates the suction, so that fluid or other matter can be sucked up the working end of the instrument. Unlike in open (i.e. non-laparoscopic) surgery, in laparoscopic surgery the assistant almost never uses the suction apparatus.

### Diathermy

This is similar to the diathermy used in open surgery, with the obvious exception that the working part is mounted at the end of a laparoscopic instrument. There are several different designs, but it commonly takes the form of a simple L-shaped hook. As with the laparoscopic suction apparatus (see above), the assistant very rarely uses the laparoscopic diathermy. However, the tip of the instrument often accumulates a deposit of carbonised material, and you may be asked to remove this, because it interferes with the operation (see p. 79). The hook is made of quite soft wire, so it is easy to bend it out of shape if your cleaning endeavours are over-enthusiastic.

## Instruments on the scrub nurse's trolley

Essentially, these are similar to instruments used in open surgery, except that their operating parts are usually smaller, and mounted on the end of long slim shafts to enable them to pass through the laparoscopic ports. Some have a ratchet mechanism on the handle.

## Driving the camera

Often, this task is referred to as *holding* the camera. This word suggests an entirely passive role, as though the assistant were merely a biological tripod. The author therefore prefers the term *driving* the camera to emphasise the active participation of a good camera-operator. If operations could be done better by simply resting the camera in an inert tripod, there would be no need for a human assistant. Indeed, robots designed for this purpose and equipped with voice-recognition technology have existed for years, but at the time of writing, have failed to gain widespread popularity. In the author's opinion, this is probably because of a combination of factors, such as expense and imperfect voice-recognition, but also at least partly because of their passivity. And perhaps because you can't chat to them about your golf handicap.

At certain points during a laparoscopic operation, the surgeon may take the camera from you and drive it him or herself. This particularly tends to occur at stages of the operation where the scope needs to move around a lot, for example, during initial inspection of the abdominal cavity or during irrigation. Do not be offended by this. Almost always, the surgeon is not confiscating the camera from you on grounds of incompetence. Rather, it is simply easier for you both if the surgeon drives the camera at this point of the operation, rather than give a rapid torrent of continuous instructions ('up a bit, left–left–left–left, stop, in a bit', etc.).

Some points of laparoscopic camera-driving technique include:

### Use the correct grip (see Figure 12.2)

Hold the camera body and not the focus ring (arrowed). Only small movements are needed to adjust the focus, so if you grasp the camera by the focus ring, you may inadvertently cause the picture to lose focus. Instead, place your fingers so that you can reach forward to adjust the focus if needed, by twisting the focus ring with index finger and thumb, as shown. If you have very small hands, you may not be able to do this. In that case, simply adjust the focus with your other hand if it is free, or ask the scrub nurse to do it for you.

## Watch the screen continuously

Taking one's eyes off the road is ill-advised when driving a car, and almost as ill-advised when driving a laparoscopic camera. While the surgeon is operating, try to watch the monitor screen continuously. However, just as it is sometimes necessary to glance away from the road for a moment when driving (e.g. to glance at the speedometer), it is sometimes necessary to glance away from the monitor screen (e.g. to activate the lens irrigator). Ensure that such glances *are* glances, and not extended surveys. It is surprising how much the picture can wander off the site of the action, if you look away for a few moments.

## Frame the picture (see Figure 12.3)

Like a good photographer or television camera operator, try to frame the picture on the screen appropriately. Try to strike a balance between too close and too distant. Too close, and the surgeon will have difficulty bringing instruments into the picture from 'off-screen'. Furthermore, the scope lens will quickly become dirtied by smoke and specks of blood from the operation itself. Too distant, and the surgeon will not be able to see what he or she is doing.

Keep the action (i.e. the area where the surgeon is operating), in the centre of the screen, and not off to one side. A simple guide is to keep the tip of the main operating instrument (which is almost always the one in the surgeon's dominant hand) in the centre of the screen.

An exception to this rule occurs when the surgeon is inserting working ports through the abdominal wall (see Figure 12.4). Here, the sharp tip of the port's trochar will usually enter the peritoneal cavity suddenly, when the tissues give way under the surgeon's pushing. Before this occurs, try to anticipate where the trochar will enter. Initially, do this by inspecting the exterior part of the port and estimating roughly where its tip will be. Aim the scope at a corresponding point on the peritoneum. Pulling the camera back for a broad 'panoramic' view will make this easier. Allow for the port's oblique passage through a thick abdominal wall.

The peritoneum is quite elastic, so before the trochar enters the peritoneal cavity, it will usually raise a little pyramid of peritoneum. Look for this little pyramid, and keep it towards the side of the screen, with its apex pointing towards the centre of the screen. In this way, as the trochar point suddenly enters, the surgeon can see where best to aim it, to avoid injury to structures such as bowel and liver.

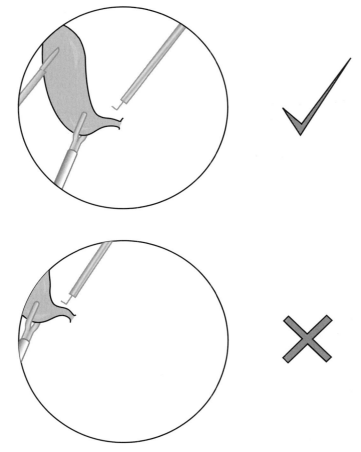

**Figure 12.3** Correct framing of a laparoscopic picture. In this example, the operation is a laparoscopic cholecystectomy. The site of surgical action (i.e. the operating surgeon's hook instrument) is in the centre of the screen in the correct view, but almost out of the picture in the incorrect view.

At all times, keep the foreground of the picture as clear as reasonably possible. In particular, try to avoid filling the foreground with a large area of anything light-coloured, such as omentum or the interior of the instrument port. A light-coloured foreground causes glare, and the camera will automatically adjust for this by making the background (where the surgeon is operating) dim and difficult to see.

If it mysteriously becomes difficult to frame the picture correctly, with limited space between the roof and the floor of the operative field, this is usually a sign that the pneumoperitoneum has disappeared. When this occurs, the peritoneal space collapses in on the operative field and laparoscope. This is sometimes

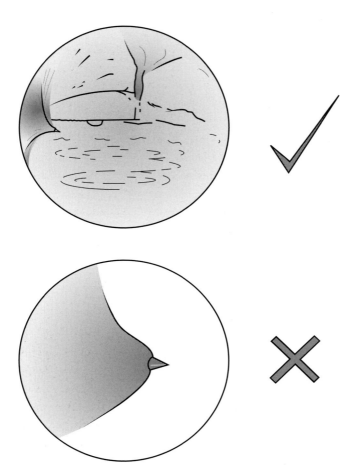

**Figure 12.4**  Top: Correct framing of a laparoscopic picture during the insertion of working ports. Note how a 'panoramic' view is used (by pulling the camera back). The sharp tip of the trochar is at the edge (not the centre) of the screen, so that structures beyond it are visible, and can be avoided as the trochar enters. Bottom: incorrect view. The camera is too close, with the trochar tip in the centre of the field. The surgeon is unable to tell whether it is safe to insert the port, because as the trochar enters, its tip may dart out of view.

known as 'Indiana Jones phenomenon' as it recalls a famous scene in the movie 'Indiana Jones and the Temple of Doom'. In this scene, the stone walls and ceiling of a special room in an ancient building slowly close in, with the intention of crushing the unwelcome occupant, the hero Indiana Jones.

Indiana Jones phenomenon is easy to recognise when a broad 'panoramic' view is in use, but it may not be obvious if it occurs during close-up work. It is caused either by not enough gas entering the peritoneal cavity (e.g. because the $CO_2$ cylinder is empty) or too much gas leaving (usually via a leak at a port or port-site).

## Avoid unnecessary movement

While the surgeon is dissecting, or performing some other important manoeuvre, keep camera movements small or keep still altogether. Aim to make any major re-adjustments to your picture, only while the surgeon is doing something that does not depend on the best possible image (e.g. exchanging the dissecting instruments). This is also the best time to clean the scope-tip.

While it is important to provide the surgeon with the best view possible, and the author prefers the term 'driving' the camera to 'holding' it, this does not mean that the camera should be continuously in motion. Indeed, continuous motion can cause a sensation of seasickness to the surgeon and anyone else watching the screen. Rather, it is better to provide the surgeon with a still picture, but adjust it to another still picture whenever necessary.

In anything but the shortest operations, you will need to change your posture to stay comfortable. This will inevitably cause the picture to wobble slightly. Therefore, if possible, avoid making big shifts in your posture during important manoeuvres.

## 'Zoom in' or 'Zoom out' when it is helpful

When the surgeon is placing instruments in through the ports, zoom out by pulling the camera back a few centimetres to give a 'panoramic' view. Keep the operative site in the centre, while showing the inner tip of the port (through which the instrument will soon emerge) in one corner of the screen. As the instrument tip appears in the port, zoom in again by following the instrument back to the operative site. This makes it much easier for the surgeon to guide the instrument tips to the operative site; otherwise, it is surprisingly easy for him or her to steer them off to an unknown fate elsewhere.

It is almost never useful to zoom further out than the inner tip of the port. Zooming out further than that point, simply shows the inside of the port, and not more of the operative field. If you have withdrawn the scope to that point, but you still feel a wider angle of view is necessary, you can achieve this by pulling the port itself partially out through the abdominal wall. This is possible because the port's inner end normally protrudes several centimetres beyond the peritoneum, into the abdominal cavity. Therefore, the extent to which it can be pulled out depends on the length of the port and the thickness of the patient's abdominal wall. Pulling the port back must be done carefully, to avoid pulling it partly or even completely out of the abdominal wall. Re-inserting a port is usually quite simple, but it wastes time and the surgeon will probably be annoyed at having to do so.

Some of the newer cameras have a zoom button feature, although in the author's opinion, this feature's uses are probably limited, because it is simpler just to move the scope in or out instead. Its potential advantage is probably in situations where a close-up view is needed, but the scope cannot be inserted far enough to provide such a view (e.g. an obese patient with a very thick abdominal wall).

## Use both hands

In some operations, you may be required to hold a laparoscopic instrument with your non-camera hand. This will usually be a ratcheted instrument providing retraction on an organ. For example, in a laparoscopic cholecystectomy, you may hold an instrument that is grasping the fundus of the gallbladder in its jaws, and be asked to retract it towards the patient's head. This raises the gallbladder and liver away from the underlying tissues, exposing the operative site around the cystic duct.

Just as in 'open' surgery, the surgeon will usually pass this retracting instrument to you at the desired angle and tension, for you to maintain. In this situation, the jaws of your instrument will usually be outside the camera's field of view, and so it is easy to neglect the instrument unintentionally, as you concentrate on driving the laparoscopic camera. This results in the retraction being lost, and poor surgical access. This common error usually happens slowly and 'off-screen', so the surgeon and assistant may struggle along for some time before realising it.

Occasionally, your non-camera hand may be required to play a more active role. For example, you may accidentally release the ratchet on your retracting grasper, and be required to re-apply the grasper. Alternatively, you may be assisting at a complex laparoscopic operation (e.g. a colectomy) in which the surgical field migrates as the operation progresses, and you may therefore be required to manipulate tissues repeatedly. You may find that using laparoscopic instruments is more difficult than you imagined from observing the surgeon. Often, the instrument will not go where you want it to go, and you may suddenly feel as though you are operating via a distorting mirror. Do not be disheartened; even the most basic of laparoscopic surgical skills take time to acquire. If you are planning a career in any field that includes endoscopic surgery, you are strongly encouraged to practice the skills involved, outside the operating theatre. Most major hospitals have access to a laparoscopic surgical 'training box'.

The jaws of most laparoscopic grasping instruments can be rotated by turning a small knob near the handle. This may give the jaws a better 'angle of attack' without the need to pronate or supinate your wrist.

## Keep yourself oriented

If you become disoriented, unsure of what structure you are looking at, use the external part of the camera as a guide. That is, look at the part of the scope external to the patient's body. The direction in which it is pointing gives an obvious clue to what you are looking at.

## Keep the picture in focus (see Figure12.2)

It hardly needs to be stated that the laparoscopic picture should be in sharp focus. In most models, the focus is adjusted by twisting a ring located on the camera head next to the scope (arrowed). Once the scope is in focus, only small movements of this ring are needed to adjust it.

Laparoscopic cameras have a reasonably broad depth of field (see 'Glossary', p. 192), so that once the camera is focussed at the start of the operation, little or no adjustment is necessary. However, sometimes you might be asked to give a close-up view (e.g. during a laparoscopic cholecystectomy, when the surgeon is incising the cystic duct to allow a cholangiogram). This may cause the focus to blur. If possible, refocus by twisting the focus ring with the fingers of the hand holding the camera.

## Some common errors in driving the laparoscopic camera

### 'Batman view'*

When performing any manual task, we normally hold our heads vertically upright, and not angled to one side, torticollis-fashion. However, in laparoscopic surgery, the television camera effectively 'becomes our eyes', so tilting the camera away from vertical will also tilt the picture. Therefore, an angulated effect can easily be achieved unintentionally, by not holding the camera vertically upright.

An incorrect side-ways angled picture is sometimes called 'Batman view'. This name derives from the 1960s television series of that name, when special effects were somewhat less sophisticated than today. In Batman's fight scenes with villains, the dramatic effect was enhanced by the camera operator deliberately tilting the camera on one side.

The laparoscope can often rotate within the camera mountings. Therefore, in scopes other than 0° type (see 'the laparoscope', p. 106), a variant of Batman view will also occur if the scope rotates, even if the camera is still held perfectly vertically. Because an angled scope is normally held so that it looks downwards, holding it upside down will make it look upwards, holding it angled to the side will

---

* The terms 'Batman view' and 'Doris Day view' were originated by Mr. Martin Bruening MS FRCS(Ed.), FRACS (Consultant General Surgeon, The Queen Elizabeth Hospital, Adelaide, South Australia) and Mr. Michael Eaton MD FRACS (Consultant Breast-Endocrine and General Surgeon, Flinders Medical Centre, Adelaide, South Australia).

make it look sideways, and so on. In some models of scope, this problem is obvious by looking at the light cable. The light cable should project vertically from the scope. If it does not, the scope is being held at an incorrect angle. Occasionally, you can exploit this angled feature to your (and the surgeon's) advantage, by rotating the scope to give a better view.

It is not always obvious that Batman view is present, especially in close-up work. Apart from the direction in which the light cable is pointing (which applies only to angled scopes), other clues include a non-horizontal fluid level (e.g. irrigation fluid) and sometimes, angulation of the surgeon's head as he or she subconsciously tries to compensate for the camera angle.

### 'Doris Day view'*

Doris Day was a film star in the 1940s to 1960s. Close-up shots of her were often filmed in a hazy soft focus style, because she typically portrayed kindly and feminine women. However, if this effect occurs during laparoscopic surgery, the surgeon will usually complain about it in a way that is neither kindly nor especially feminine.

In Doris Day's movies, the haze was deliberately created by smearing Vaseline onto the camera lens. In laparoscopic surgery, the haze is usually caused by foreign matter on the lens of the laparoscope, or occasionally more proximally, on the lens of the camera. It is sometimes easy to guess what this foreign matter is, from the timing of when it occurs. For example, if hazing occurs soon after the scope is inserted, the foreign matter is usually water fogging on a cool lens-tip in the warm humid atmosphere of the pneumoperitoneum. This can be prevented by warming the scope tip, either before inserting it (e.g. by placing the warm palm of your hand against the tip) or after insertion by gently wiping it against the viscera (see below).

Other causes of haze on the lens include particles of matter sprayed from the operation site (e.g. smoke or specks of blood). Smears of fat or fluid can appear on the lens, arising from brushing against organs inside the peritoneum, or from small pieces of debris trapped in the port itself.

It can be difficult to judge when it is appropriate to clean the lens. Some surgeons insist on a very clear sharp picture at all times, while others prefer to tolerate a degree of Doris Day view rather than interrupt the operation to get rid of it. Therefore, always ask the surgeon before cleaning the lens. Depending on the cause, the following manoeuvres can be used.

Some scopes are provided with an irrigating sleeve. As the name suggests, this squirts water onto the lens, like the similar feature that cleans the windscreen of a car. It is usually highly effective. If this device is not being used, or is ineffective, you can wipe the lens gently on some nearby tissue, such as liver or omentum. If this does not work, you may have to remove the scope from the port, clean the lens and dip it in an antifog solution.

Sometimes the scope is removed and cleaned, only to become hazy again immediately on re-insertion into the port. This is usually caused either by water condensation (see above) or by tissue debris accumulating within the port itself and contaminating the lens on insertion. Obviously, this latter situation can only be corrected by cleaning the port. Sometimes, simply inserting the corner of a clean pack into the port, and rotating it is enough, but often the port must be partly dismantled.

# 13 Neurosurgery

**Amal Abou-Hamden** MBBS

Department of Neurosurgery, Royal Adelaide Hospital, North Terrace, Adelaide, South Australia

**Steve Santoreneos** MBBS FRACS

Department of Neurosurgery, Royal Adelaide Hospital, North Terrace, Adelaide, South Australia

## Introduction

Nerve tissue is delicate, easily damaged, and has a poor capacity for repair. This is especially true of the cortex and spinal cord, and injury to these structures may obviously have devastating consequences. Therefore, it is extremely important that when you are assisting at neurosurgical operations, you handle the tissues gently, if at all.

## ■ Equipment

As in other areas of surgery, it is helpful to be familiar with the equipment you will be using. In cranial neurosurgical procedures, this equipment will often include the Mayfield skull clamp, which is a table-mounted instrument designed to hold the head firmly in position. It does so by means of three pins which are fixed to the bony skull vault. Usually the surgeon will apply the pins and then ask you to tighten the clamps in position while he or she positions the head.

The Greenberg retractor is another table-mounted instrument, commonly used in intra-cranial surgery. It can be fitted with a variety of tissue-retracting blades. If the surgeon asks you to loosen one of these blades, be very clear on which blade you are to loosen. The blade may be very near a critical structure, such as an aneurysm, which may rupture as you remove the blade.

Specialised tables are normally used for spinal surgery (e.g. the Jackson table and the Andrews table).

In some centres, the Stealth® system may be used. Briefly, this system uses complex computer imaging to localise anatomical (and pathological) structures with great accuracy – often within less than 1 mm. Obviously, it is important not to lean on the frame of such a precision instrument.

# ■ Surgical access

Although there is large variety of different intra-cranial operations, from the assistant's viewpoint, the principles of many of them are similar. In particular, the steps required to enter the skull vault are similar.

The soft tissues overlying the skull contain nerves that can sometimes be injured by careless retraction. For example, retraction of the temporalis muscle in a myocutaneous scalp flap with a Raike retractor should be done gently, to avoid injury to the frontalis branch of the facial nerve. Care should also be exercised when retracting the scalp over the supraorbital nerve region. A Langenbeck retractor is preferred in this location.

Once the soft tissues have been retracted, the bony skull is the next layer encountered. The surgeon will usually enter the skull by drilling it with a 'burr', which is a drill-bit with an approximately spherical shape. Just like when using a household drill, the process of drilling the skull generates heat. A small amount of heat is beneficial, as it helps secure haemostasis at the bone edges. However, excessive heat can easily be generated, and is potentially harmful to the tissues. Drilling also generates bone dust, which can float off into the surrounding surgical field.

The two problems of excess heat and floating bone dust can both be prevented by irrigating the drill site with saline. You will be provided with a syringe filled with saline, for this purpose. Some surgeons prefer that you only irrigate when they stop drilling, while others prefer gentle continuous irrigation (in drops).

Sometimes a router is used to elevate a craniotomy flap; if so, you should use both irrigation and suction to keep the wound free of bone dust. If possible, irrigate slightly in front of the advancing tip of the router with the syringe in one hand, and suck up the bone dust–saline mixture behind it with the other.

After removal of the bone flap, gently irrigate the dura to enable the surgeon to identify any significant bleeding points which need to be coagulated. The surgeon will then open the dura mater. He or she will make the first opening in the dura with a sharp hook or a blade, then complete the dural opening with a fine toothed forceps and dural scissors. You need to maintain the surgeon's visibility by either gentle irrigation or suction at the leading edge of the dural incision.

Working under the light of the microscope can contribute to the drying of tissues. Therefore, once the brain is on view, keep it and the vessels moist by irrigating with warm Ringer's solution (using the bulb irrigator or 20–50 ml syringe), particularly when the surgeon is dissecting arteries (e.g. in aneurysm surgery).

# ■ Use of suckers

As mentioned earlier, nerve tissue is easily injured and has a poor capacity for repair. It is so delicate that direct contact with the suction device can easily cause injury. Therefore, when operating on the cerebral cortex or spinal cord, fluids such as blood and cerebrospinal fluid are not suctioned directly off the tissues. Instead, special swabs known as 'cottonoid patties' (or usually, simply 'patties') are used. These are squares of woven cotton-like material, about as big as a fingernail. To lessen the chances of such a small object being lost in the surgical field, they have a string attached to one corner. To suck up fluid with this method, place the pattie on a convenient area, and press the tip of the sucker gently against it. Fluid is then sucked through the pattie into the sucker, protecting the underlying tissues from direct contact with the sucker.

Use your thumb to control the amount of suction. If you're operating on cortex or nerve roots, roll your thumb off the hole in the sucker to decrease suction and/or be prepared to squeeze the suction tubing. You need to be prepared to do this immediately when the surgeon says 'squeeze the sucker'.

# ■ Retraction

It is always important to be conscious of the amount of pressure exerted when retracting any tissue, but this is of critical importance in neural tissue. You may be asked to hold a brain retractor for a long time; it is not uncommon for neuro-surgical operations to last for eight hours or more. Ensure that you rest your hand on a nearby, safe surface and retract gently. When holding the retractor for prolonged periods, the tendency is for the angle of the retractor to change and result in 'digging' into the cortex and/or white matter, so you must be constantly mindful of the position of your retractor.

If the operation is a resection of a tumour, you may be asked to hold the tumour up with tumour-holding forceps. In this case, avoid the natural tendency to pull up. You are only holding the tumour up to facilitate deeper dissection of the tumour by the surgeon. It is not your job to 'remove the tumour', and excessive traction puts deep vessels on a stretch and at risk of serious bleeding. Again, you may be asked to do this for hours at a time, so rest your hand.

In spinal surgery (e.g. microdiscectomy), you may be asked to retract a nerve root medially whilst the surgeon performs the discectomy. Avoid injury to the nerve root, by only retracting on it gently, and secondly by sliding out the retractor gently.

# ■ Assisting using the microscope (see also p. 126 and 154)

It is worth familiarizing yourself briefly with the relevant aspects of the microscope before the start of the operation. Always make sure that your eyepiece is oriented correctly at the beginning of the case. The first time you may be required to introduce any instruments under the microscope may be to use a sucker during an intra-operative rupture of an aneurysm, and that is not the time to orientate yourself.

Always inform the surgeon when you need to adjust your eyepiece and avoid doing this at critical parts of the surgery.

# ■ Shunt surgery (see also 'prosthetic materials', p. 90)

It is best to double-glove during these procedures, and to use non-powdered gloves. Avoid handling the shunt tubing directly with your hands; always use protected forceps instead.

## SUGGESTED FURTHER READING

Greenberg MSS. *Handbook of Neurosurgery* (5th edition). Thieme, Lakeland, Florida USA 2001.

Connolly Jr ES, McKhann GM II, Huang J and Choudhri T. *Fundamentals of Operative Techniques in Neurosurgery*. Thieme, New York, USA 2002.

Kaye AH and Black P. *Operative Neurosurgery*. Churchill Livingstone, London 2000.

# 14 Obstetric and gynaecological surgery

**Angelique Swart** BSc (Hons) BMBS Dip RANZCOG

Department of Obstetrics and Gynaecology, Flinders Medical Centre, Flinders Drive, Bedford Park, Adelaide, South Australia

**Elinor Atkinson** MBBS FRANZCOG

Department of Obstetrics and Gynaecology, Flinders Medical Centre, Flinders Drive, Bedford Park, Adelaide South Australia

## ■ Obstetric operations

The Obstetric operation essentially refers to a Caesarean Section (CS). This operation is usually a joy to perform and is most often associated with a positive outcome. However it can be very stressful, as events can suddenly turn for the worse, with two or more lives at stake. Also, unlike most other operations, CS often must be performed urgently to minimise foetal distress. Consequently, most surgeons performing CS greatly appreciate an assistant who has some prior understanding of the operation. It is therefore strongly recommended that you familiarise yourself with the steps of the operation beforehand, either by reference to an operative text (see 'suggested further reading', p. 123) or by discussion with a senior colleague.

The hazard of fainting in the operating theatre is particularly real at CS. This is because the temperature of the operating theatre is deliberately raised, to reduce the risk of hypothermia to the infant (see 'If you feel faint' p. 8 for further advice).

Before scrubbing, it is recommended that you don a waterproof gown or apron (see p. 36), to protect yourself from blood and amniotic fluid.

During the operation, the woman lies on the operating table on her back. A right-handed surgeon will almost always stand on the woman's right side. You, the assistant, will stand opposite the surgeon (i.e. almost always on the woman's left side).

As for most operations, a standard skin preparation and draping with sterile towels is done. The surgeon incises the skin and spreads the rectus muscles in the midline. The peritoneal cavity is entered and the bladder is reflected, revealing the uterus. As the assistant, it is important at this stage to maintain steady retraction of the bladder. Usually this is done with the Doyen retractor.

To maximise room for delivery of the infant, it is also helpful to maintain traction on the rectus sheath and abdominal wall in the cephalad direction (i.e. towards the woman's head). A Langenbeck's retractor is usually used for this purpose. As the surgeon delivers the infant's head, gently remove the bladder retractor in an upwards direction (i.e. towards the ceiling). It is important to do this carefully, to avoid bumping the infant on the head. Once the surgeon delivers the head, place one hand firmly on the uterine fundus and push the infant's body out, by pushing in the same direction as a uterine contraction. That is, push the fundus towards the mother's feet, and not downwards into her epigastrium. Pushing towards the epigastrium is ineffective, and is a mistake which assistants commonly make.

Once the infant is delivered, cut the cord while the surgeon holds the infant. Place a clamp a few centimetres from the umbilicus, and 'milk the cord' of blood by gently squeezing its contained blood towards the placenta. Then place a second clamp 2–3 cm away from the first, towards the placenta. If cord gases are to be taken a third clamp may be placed a further 10–15 cm along the cord, towards the placenta. A common mistake by novice assistants is to cut the cord without first ensuring that the clamp is firmly placed on either side, resulting in cord blood splattering around the room.

When the uterus, peritoneum and rectus sheath are being closed, assist by holding ('following') the suture material with your right hand, while at the same time retracting the overlying tissue layers (e.g. the rectus sheath and bladder) with the left hand (see p. 88 for the correct way to 'follow' a suture). This is a skill that takes experience to develop. Ensure that you never cross your hands or obstruct the surgeon's view of the operative field.

When the surgeon is closing the rectus sheath, use a Langenbeck retractor to expose the edges of the sheath. This is especially helpful when the surgeon is placing the first suture. As closure progresses, try not to retract too hard, as this makes it more difficult to appose the two edges of the rectus sheath, and risks strangulating the tissues.

## SUGGESTED FURTHER READING

O'Grady JP *et al*. Caesarean delivery. In *Operative Obstetrics* (Chapter 11) eds JP O'Grady, ML Gimovsky and CJ McIlhargie. Williams and Wilkins, Sydney, 1995, pp. 239–264.

# ■ Gynaecological operations

Gynaecological operations at which an assistant is usually present, include hysterectomy (via the abdominal or vaginal approach), vaginal repairs and laparoscopic procedures. Assisting at laparoscopic procedures is discussed elsewhere, in Chapter 12, (p. 103).

If you are a trainee assisting at a gynaecological operation, the gynaecologist will often ask you to learn, or improve your skills at, vaginal examinations, by examining the patient after she is anaesthetised. This is obviously a less stressful way for the patient to undergo such an examination. However, it is very important that you obtain permission from the patient to do so, and that such permission is obtained before the patient has received sedative medication.

During vaginal surgery, the patient is almost always lying on her back with her legs raised, flexed at the hip and knee. The legs are supported in this position either by simple canvas stirrups, or by specially designed cradles, sometimes known as Lloyd–Davies stirrups. The surgeon either sits or stands between the patient's legs. Therefore, when assisting at vaginal operations, you will usually stand beside one of the patient's legs (more commonly the left). This means you will have to reach over the patient's leg in order to hold instruments such as haemostats or 'clips', vaginal wall retractors and one-handled Sims retractors. It can be difficult to do this while still maintaining good posture, and avoiding back discomfort or injury. This is especially so if the patient's legs are supported in simple stirrups instead of Lloyd–Davies stirrups.

Try to ensure that only your arms (and not your trunk) lean over the patient's leg. Keep your back straight, and avoid hunching forwards.

Avoid leaning on the patient's leg excessively, especially when this compresses the leg against the stirrups' supporting pole. Occasionally, this can cause post-operative leg pain, which besides being uncomfortable for the patient, can require investigation to differentiate it from deep-vein thrombosis. Although it is rare, compartment syndrome has occurred from muscular injury by this mechanism. If you are lucky, the surgeon may use a special retractor (e.g. 'Lonestar') and clips to reduce the assistant's need to hold several instruments simultaneously.

### SUGGESTED FURTHER READING

Rock JA and Jones III HW (eds). *Te Linde's Operative Gynecology* (9th edition). Lippincott Williams and Wilkins, Philadelphia, USA, 2003.

# Ophthalmic surgery 15

**Graham Fraenkel** BMBS FRANZCO FRACS

Cataract and Laser Surgicentre, North Terrace, Adelaide, South Australia

Assisting in ophthalmology has a different culture to assisting in many other surgical subspecialties. Gone are the Wellington boots, the muscle-seizing retractors, the gurgling suction devices and the general banter that progresses under general anaesthetic in a happy operating theatre.

These are replaced with microscopes, smaller areas of Betadine, often rapid turnover of patients, and a respect for the fact that for most operations, the patient is well awake. Ophthalmic surgery is performed more and more in specialised day surgical facilities, rather than in major general hospitals. Patients are therefore seen by the assistant post-operatively less and less, as this usually takes place in the surgeon's outpatients or rooms, and less and less on the ward.

The spectrum of ophthalmic operations at which you may assist, varies from cataract surgery to complex procedures such as anterior reconstructive surgery, involving delicate suturing of the sclera, cornea, iris, and perhaps intraocular lens, vitreo-retinal surgery, extraocular muscle surgery, and oculoplastic surgery.

By far the commonest ophthalmic operation is cataract surgery. Indeed, it is the world's commonest prosthetic operation. However, the proportion of cataract operations being performed with an assistant is rapidly decreasing, because improvements in design of the prosthetic lenses have made the operation simpler to perform. The most common assistant at cataract surgery is a future cataract surgeon honing his or her skills.

## ■ Pre-operative preparation

The surgeon may expect you to procure the intraocular lens of a particular type and power as stated on the operating list. As there is no greater cause for ophthalmic litigation than the insertion of the wrong intraocular lens, this is a job you should gently try to refuse if you are not familiar with it. If you are not but the surgeon is insistent, seek guidance from experienced theatre staff. In most institutions, a selection of lenses will be sitting on a convenient shelf.

The next step is to check whether it is the patient's left or right eye that is to be operated on. Then, nursing or technical staff will instil drops into the eye, to dilate the pupil. The patient is then ushered into the pre-anaesthetic area, where preparation of the operative site often begins with the application of povidone–iodine solution ('Betadine') to the conjunctival sac, eyelashes and surrounding skin. The Betadine is half strength (5%) and contains no alcohol. Be careful not to use full strength Betadine or alcohol-based antiseptics, as they can injure the eye.

Once the patient is in theatre the Betadine is re-applied. While it dries, you should check that your side of the operating microscope (known as the 'assistant branch' of the microscope), is adjusted correctly for you. Specifically, adjust the interpupillary distance, dioptric power and tilt of the eyepieces for comfortable viewing. Some assistant branches will have rings for adjusting the orientation of the image. If in doubt, summon the courage to ask your surgeon for assistance. This wise investment in humility will prevent the greater loss of face which you will feel, if the microscope needs to be adjusted once the procedure is underway. A particularly embarrassing error is to have the image in your eyepieces oriented incorrectly (e.g. upside down). This will quickly become obvious, because your attempts to manoeuvre your instruments will have the opposite effect to that desired, both on your instruments and on the surgeon's demeanor.

You should then scrub, gown and glove in the normal manner (see p. 36). Once gowned and gloved, you may be asked to assist in draping. Most ophthalmic surgeons use a special plastic drape, designed to keep the eyelids and eyelashes out of the surgical field. You can provide specific assistance here, by holding back the eyelids and lashes, while the surgeon applies the drape. This is normally done with instruments resembling long cotton buds, and known as reversed orange sticks. This is an important task, because an eyelash falling into the wound is the most common cause of post-operative infection.

Once the procedure is underway, your main role will be to keep the cornea moist so that it maintains transparency for the surgeon's optimum view. Do this by periodically instilling a drop of irrigation fluid (balanced salt solution) gently into the eye. Normally, the eye hydrates itself with only a thin film of tears. If you instil too much solution, it can injure the corneal epithelium. Therefore, the fewer drops of you use to achieve hydration of the cornea, the better.

Otherwise, from the assistant's viewpoint, the operation is about as simple as could be found. The only retractor (the lid speculum) is self-retaining. No sutures or clips are used in modern cataract surgery. Loading the intraocular lens into the appropriate delivery device is a specialised procedure and different for each lens type, and so is normally performed by the surgeon or the scrub nurse.

The patient will usually be quite wide awake, and so caution will need to be exercised. The usual operating room banter will have to be laid aside, and any unexpected events or operative mishaps met with silence.

However, not all patients are wide awake; sedation is used in some. In this situation, try to keep the patient's behaviour under surveillance. Confused patients have been known to rouse suddenly, and raise their hands to remove the eyelid retractor, with potentially disastrous consequences. A quick response, grasping the patient's hand through the drape and preventing this unsolicited surgical assistance, will be appreciated by the surgeon. Similarly, you should also warn the surgeon if you think the patient has fallen asleep. Ophthalmic surgery requires the surgeon's full concentration. Often he or she will be simultaneously operating with both hands and feet (much like an organ player), concentrating on small movements in the operative field, as well as listening to the sounds made by the various specialised machines as they indicate levels of suction and cutting. Therefore, the surgeon can become quite unaware of the patient's level of consciousness, and will be relying on you and the anaesthetist to alert him or her to any problems looming outside the operative field.

In contrast to the undemanding nature of assisting at most cataract surgery, assisting at vitreo-retinal surgery can potentially occupy the opposite extreme. The author has personally assisted at a seven-hour procedure, for the majority of which a lens had to be delicately balanced on the cornea to provide the surgeon with a view of the posterior chamber of the eye, while maintaining hydration of the cornea and preparing silicon fluids for infusion into the eye through an assemblage of three-way taps. As the retina is derived from neuroectoderm, the analogy with neurosurgery would appear appropriate.

Several highly specialised instruments are used in this field. They include cryotherapy probes for retinal repairs, probes for transilluminating the retina, and indirect ophthalmoscopes for illuminating the ocular interior. Your role will be to assist the surgeon in locating and closing retinal breaks, and performing the process of vitrectomy. In this latter procedure, the intraocular vitreous jelly is cut into small pieces and sucked out via an automated instrument. Filling the ocular volume afterwards with gas or specialised liquids is performed via electric or hand driven pumps.

Ophthalmic instruments are particularly delicate and expensive. They need to be handled carefully to avoid damaging them. As with all surgical instruments, you should only use them for the specific purpose for which they were designed.

For example, fine instruments, such as Vannas scissors (used for cutting fine sutures, such as 10/0 nylon), should not be used for cutting drapes.

Using an instrument for an incorrect purpose can also damage the delicate ocular tissues. For example, Kalibri forceps with toothed tips should not be used to handle the conjunctiva during trabeculectomy operations. This is because their tips can cause perforations of the delicate conjunctiva, which may lead to a leaking operative site.

Because the ocular tissues are so delicate, it follows that they must be handled not only with the correct instruments, but also with great gentleness. Usually, the tensions applied to ocular tissues are minimal and very precise. A 'robotic' arm is required to provide the correct and sustained tension on sutures or tissues. If you inadvertently avulse a perfect delicately crafted trabecular scleral flap, the surgeon who has just constructed it will not be your new best friend.

# Orthopaedic surgery

16

**John van Essen** BMBS FRACS

Wakefield Orthopaedic Clinic, Adelaide, South Australia
Royal Adelaide Hospital and The Queen Elizabeth Hospital, Adelaide, South Australia

## ■ Introduction

The broad field of orthopaedic surgery can be divided into elective orthopaedics and emergency (trauma) orthopaedics. In elective orthopaedics, there are two major subcategories, namely arthroscopic surgery and joint replacement surgery.

## ■ General factors related to orthopaedic surgery

### Clothing in the operating theatre (see also Chapter 3, p. 11)

In orthopaedic surgery, and in particular in joint replacement surgery, most surgeons expect that any person entering the operating theatre covers all their hair. This is usually done with a balaclava-type head cover. Sometimes 'space suits' are used; these are all-enclosing suits and helmets with an air supply pumped into them, designed to seal all the air circulating around the body of the surgeon and assistant. Eye protection should always be used, as orthopaedic surgery can be quite bloody.

### Marking the operation site (see also p. 21)

Because most orthopaedic operations are on the limbs, wrong-sided surgery is a major concern to orthopaedic surgeons. The ultimate responsibility for correct-sided surgery rests with the surgeon. However, this does not mean that the surgeon is the only member of the surgical team who is required to check which side is to be operated on. Indeed, the entire surgical team, including nursing staff, anaesthetist and you, the assistant, should be vigilant in this task. This may include checking that the patient, pre-operative notes and consent form all agree on which side is to be operated on, and checking that the patient has had a mark (e.g. an ink arrow) either prior to the entry to the theatre, or on entry into the theatre.

## Anatomical knowledge

It is very helpful for you to have revised the relevant anatomy of the joint or long bone which is to be operated on. In particular, knowledge of the dangers of injury to the associated neurovascular structures is very important. These are very specific to each site. Examples include the sciatic nerve in total hip replacement; the ulnar nerve in elbow surgery; the brachial plexus in shoulder surgery; and the tibial and peroneal nerves and popliteal vessels in knee surgery.

Because bone is tough tissue, surgeons need tough instruments such as saws and chisels to work on it, and comparatively large forces are sometimes necessary. This raises the possibility of injury to important nearby structures if they are not properly protected. When assisting at orthopaedic operations, you will commonly find that you will be using your retractors not only to retract overlying tissues and expose the operation site, but also to protect these important structures. Although the surgeon will be fully aware of this potential for injury, he or she will appreciate an extra pair of eyes watching out for it, whilst he or she concentrates on the bone. It is important that you notify the surgeon at once, if you feel that such a structure is in danger (e.g. if you notice that the surgeon's saw is close to a major artery as he or she is sawing a bone).

# Elective orthopaedic surgery: arthroscopic surgery

## ■ General tips

### Setting up

#### Positioning the patient

Space limitations do not allow a full description of correct patient positioning for all the arthroscopic operations. However, most surgeons will be very grateful for your help with this. The general principles include:

1 Where possible, apply a tourniquet to the limb proximal to the joint being operated on (e.g. apply the tourniquet to the thigh for knee arthroscopy, and to the fore-arm for wrist arthroscopy). Wrap a soft protective bandage (e.g. 'Soft-ban') beneath it. Clearly, to be effective, the tourniquet must exert a pressure that is higher than the patient's blood pressure; most surgeons routinely set it to 250 mmHg for the upper limb and 300 mmHg for the lower limb. Do not turn the tourniquet on until instructed to do so and always have the pressure gauge facing the surgeon so he or she knows the pressure.

2  To enable the surgeon to view all the surfaces inside a joint, the joint must be moved around during the operation (usually by you, the assistant, see below). Therefore, the limb must be positioned in such a way that this can occur.

3  To give the camera enough room to see inside the joint, the joint is expanded either by irrigating it with fluid or by pulling on it ('traction'), or sometimes by a combination of both. The traction may be provided by specialised machinery, such as pulley systems, or by someone (usually you) pulling on the limb. Usually, this traction is applied by pulling the joint along the long axis of the limb.

4  Like in other types of surgery, the patient is often held securely in position by cushions (bolsters) and padded devices clamped to the table. To save time, surgeons will often ask you to do this, while they scrub. Often the surgeon will tinker with your set-up; do not take this as a criticism, as the surgeon will simply be tailoring it to his or her specific preference.

### Setting up cords and cables

As in laparoscopic surgery (see p. 103) several different cords and tubes pass from the operating table to various machines 'off-table'. These tubes include the arthroscopic camera cable, light cable, diathermy lead, chondrotome cable and irrigation. Some surgeons also use a drainage tube.

Ensure you hand off the correct end of these cables and tubes; if the incorrect end is handed off, a new cable must be found, which causes unnecessary delays.

### Fluid irrigation

No matter what type of arthroscopic surgery is being performed, fluid is pumped into the joint, to expand the joint and so give enough space to allow the scope to see inside the joint. Usually this fluid is 5% glycine, but sometimes normal saline is used.

Most commonly, a hand-pump is used for the fluid. Normally it is a simple bulb type, operated by squeezing, and located about midway along the tubing. As the assistant, it is highly likely that you will be operating the pump. Sometimes a self-regulating machine is used, in which case you can rest!

Air bubbles in the fluid interfere with the surgeon's view inside the joint. Therefore, it is very important that before it is attached to the arthroscope, the irrigant tubing is primed with fluid in such a way that all air bubbles are removed. This includes evacuating air from the hand-pump (if one is used), usually by inverting it. Once the tube is primed and fluid is running through it, remember to avoid soaking the drapes by closing the valve, and leaving it closed until just before it is attached to the arthroscope.

Since fluid is pumped into the joint, it also needs to escape from the joint, and it can do this either through a drain, or by extravasation into the adjacent soft tissues. It is important to realise that the soft tissues surrounding a joint are normally enclosed in an envelope of tough fascia, forming a closed space. Consequently, if too much fluid enters this closed space, the pressure will rise, and can lead to Compartment Syndrome. This can have severe ramifications, with the death of muscle and nerve tissue in the space – obviously a most undesirable outcome.

Therefore, at all times you must be constantly aware of the amount of fluid that has been pumped into the joint space. Regulate the fluid flow by gently pinching the inflow tubing between thumb and forefinger, and only using enough fluid to maintain clear vision. Usually, only intermittent pumping is needed. A common mistake made by assistants is to use a gorilla-like grip, with the type of continuous pumping which one would normally associate with milking a cow. This is not desirable; farm hands need not apply. With large joints (such as the hip, knee and shoulder) pumping needs to be performed only occasionally, while for the smaller joints (ankle, elbow and wrist) little or no pumping is usually required.

## Handling of instruments

Sometimes the scrub nurse will be unable to pass instruments directly to the surgeon, and it is simply more practical for you to do so. Also, sometimes you may need to hold on to instruments that the surgeon is using frequently, rather than handing them back and forth repeatedly to the scrub nurse. Ideally, you should pass instruments to the surgeon handle-first, and with the tips as close as possible to the portal into which the surgeon will be feeding the instrument.

## Holding the scope

To help orient themselves within the three-dimensional space of a joint, most orthopaedic surgeons use a technique known as 'triangulation'. Briefly, this means that they hold the camera in their left hand, an operating instrument in their right, and carefully watch the instruments on the screen monitor. The camera, instrument and monitor therefore make up the three elements of a triangle. Note that in contrast to laparoscopic surgery, the surgeon (not the assistant) normally drives the camera in arthroscopic surgery.

However, for technical reasons (e.g. the need to re-adjust the position of the limb or the operating instrument), the surgeon may sometimes ask you to hold the camera. This means that, in a sense, one element of the triangle is removed, and the surgeon can become 'lost in space' if you do not keep the camera, and therefore the image on the monitor, as still as possible.

# ■ Arthroscopy of larger joints

## Shoulder arthroscopy

Shoulder arthroscopy is performed in two main positions, namely the 'beach chair' position and the lateral position. In the beach chair position, no traction is used (apart from gravity on the arm), whereas in the lateral position, traction is applied by a system of pulleys at the end of the bed. In either case your main role as the assistant will probably be to supplement the traction. In the 'beach chair' position this will usually be simply pulling the arm down towards the floor, while in the lateral position you may be asked to raise the arm towards the ceiling.

## Knee arthroscopy

In virtually all cases, the patient will be supine. Some surgeons use a variation in which the leg is free to flex to 90° over the end of the bed. To save time, some surgeons like to scrub, while you position the patient.

Once the arthroscopy is under way, the surgeon will normally need little assistance (apart from monitoring the irrigation) as he or she assesses the patellofemoral and medial compartments. Only after the surgeon has moved across the intercondylar notch area into the lateral compartment will your assistance be required. At this point, the surgeon will lift the leg up into a cross legged (figure of 4) position, at which point you should grasp the leg at the ankle and keep it in place. It is imperative to do this gently, as the scope can easily fall out of the joint space. The surgeon may switch back and forth between lateral and medial compartments at any time, so be prepared to reposition the leg at any time.

# ■ Arthroscopy of smaller joints

The arthroscopes used in these joints are usually shorter and smaller in diameter than those used in larger joints, to prevent excess leverage on the joint. Also, because the joint is smaller, you must be careful not to instil too much irrigation fluid. Surgeons sometimes use a small needle (e.g. 23 gauge) to locate smaller joints, and may ask you to withdraw the needle as they make their skin incision.

### Ankle arthroscopy

Like shoulder arthroscopy, ankle arthroscopy can be performed with or without traction equipment. When it is performed without such equipment, you may be called upon to act as the traction device. Do this by pulling on the foot towards the sole, in an effort to distract the ankle joint.

### Elbow arthroscopy

This can be performed either with the patient in a lateral position with the arm over an arm rest, or with the patient supine with the hand suspended by finger trap traction. In the lateral position it is surprisingly easy for the surgeon to become disoriented between the medial and lateral aspects of the joint, and this could potentially result in ulnar nerve injury. It is helpful for you to warn the surgeon if you feel the surgeon is close to the nerve. (Remember that the ulnar nerve is on the medial side.)

### Wrist arthroscopy

Again, you may be required to act as a counter-traction device by pushing on the upper arm, while the fingers are suspended in finger trap traction.

# Elective orthopaedic surgery: major joint replacement
## ■ General principles

### Preparation

Most companies that make prosthetic joints provide accompanying booklets in the packaging, describing the surgical technique in some detail. Ideally, you should aim to study these prior to assisting at such operations to help with anticipating the steps involved.

Infection of a foreign object implanted anywhere in the body is usually difficult to treat, and a dreaded complication of any operation where a prosthesis (such as a joint replacement) is inserted (see 'Prosthetic materials', p. 90). Furthermore, established infection in bone (even without an implanted foreign body) is also difficult to treat. Therefore, it follows that infection of an implant within bone is a particularly bad combination of events. Consequently, meticulous attention to sterility is of extreme importance in joint replacement surgery.

It is very important that at any stage during the operation you suspect that you have breached sterile conditions, you must immediately identify this to the surgeon and change both your gown and your gloves. It is better to have changed several times than to have risked any chance of infection into the joint replacement.

## Draping

As you paint the skin and drape up, the surgeon and yourself will usually each be wearing two pairs of gloves. Once draping has been performed, and the wound-site has been sealed with a wound protector (e.g. 'Betadine Opsite'), remove and discard your outer pair of gloves. Do this in a sterile manner, being careful not to contaminate the inner gloves by touching the 'contact areas' of the outer glove. Then put on a new pair of outer gloves.

## Setting up

Following the draping, there follows quite a deal of activity, setting up and passing off tubes and cords, including suction, diathermy and irrigation (pulse lavage). The above instruments are normally placed in a receiver attached to the drapes. To prevent them slipping off the table, the instruments' attached lines should also be clipped to the drapes at an appropriate length, that is outside the operative field, but within easy reach of both the surgeon and the operation site.

## Intra-operatively

Most orthopaedic surgeons use a special type of irrigation system, which delivers pulsatile flow and is known as 'pulse lavage'. During the operation, you should aim to use this in combination with the suction, to keep the operative field clear of blood and bone debris. This is especially so, while the surgeon is reaming out the bone, preparing the bed in which the artificial joint will sit. If possible, use the pulse lavage in one hand, and the suction in the other. However, this is sometimes not possible, as you must sometimes support the limb.

The cement used in joint replacement surgery hardens very quickly: typically it only remains soft enough to be worked for a few minutes. For some operations (e.g. total knee replacement), this means that a critical time-balancing act occurs: before the cement hardens, several components of the prosthesis must all be placed in their proper positions, seated correctly, and all the excess cement removed. It is crucial that you provide the surgeon with adequate exposure at this time, by retracting appropriately. The surgeon will work furiously at this time, aware that when the cement hardens there is no turning back if components are in the wrong place!

Immediately after joint replacement surgery, new joints (particularly hips and shoulders) are vulnerable to dislocation if not handled carefully. Therefore, at the end of the operation, it is especially important that either you or the surgeon stays with the patient to supervise the transfer from the operating table to ward bed. Often, this will be your job because the surgeon will depart to write up the operative note. In this case, ensure that clamps are removed carefully, and that the limb is kept positioned according to the surgeon's instructions.

## ■ Tips for assisting at specific operations

### Total hip replacement

This may be done by either an anterior or posterior approach. The patient usually lies on his or her side (lateral position) but it can also be done from the supine position, depending on the surgeon's preference. Often you will be asked to lift the leg, while the surgical site is being prepared with antiseptic paint. A common mistake made by assistants at this stage, is to allow the operation site to become contaminated. This occurs when the lateral position is being used, and the assistant (holding the foot), is asked to abduct the leg towards the ceiling but fails to maintain external rotation of the limb. External rotation (i.e. pointing the toes towards the ceiling) locks the knee in full extension, and if this is not done, the knee flexes, collapsing down and the painted area touches an unsterile area of the bed.

During the operation, after the femoral head has been dislocated from the hip joint, it can become quite loose and floppy and may even roll off the operating table. Prevent this from occurring by standing close to the table. If you are endowed with a large abdomen, you will be able to control the movement of the leg better.

A key point of assisting at this operation arises when the surgeon is preparing the femoral canal for insertion of the prosthesis: you must hold the limb rock-steady at this point. This helps the surgeon to orient the prosthesis properly, and a few degrees either way can mean the difference between a secure, snug-fitting hip replacement and a dislocating useless lump of metal.

### Total knee replacement

A key point for the assistant occurs early in the operation. The incision used is usually a midline incision with a medial para-patellar approach. Once the patella is everted, the knee is gently flexed up. A common mistake is for an over-zealous assistant to force the knee vigorously up into flexion. This can result in either avulsion of the patellar tendon or a fracture of the femoral condyle, neither of which the surgeon wishes to see at the start of a procedure.

Total knee replacement is an example of an operation in which you will be using your retractors not only to retract overlying tissues and expose the operation site, but also to protect important nearby structures. These structures are the collateral ligaments, the patellar tendon and the popliteal artery.

As mentioned above, in most total knee replacements, a critical step (for both you and surgeon) occurs when the bone cement is prepared and placed in the bone, because in the space of only a few minutes, all the joint components must be inserted and properly positioned and the excess cement removed.

### Post-operatively

Immediately after the operation, and particularly if a tourniquet has been used, it is important that you assess the distal blood supply to the limb. Before the patient leaves the operating theatre for the recovery room, make note of the presence of any distal pulses, and the colour of the foot or hand. Is it warm and pink with prompt capillary refill, implying satisfactory flow, or is it pale, implying no blood flow? Any concerns should be immediately notified to the surgeon.

Collect up all the X-rays and case-notes and place them on the patient's bed. This ensures everything is kept with the patient and ensures a quick turnover for the next case.

# Emergency orthopaedic surgery

Emergency orthopaedic surgery (trauma) generally implies a fracture to the bones, which may or may not involve the joints. The general principles for assisting in emergency orthopaedic surgery are very similar to those for assisting in elective orthopaedic surgery and are summarised below (for detail refer to elective orthopaedic surgery).

## ■ Positioning the patient

Prior to positioning, ask the surgeon if the Image Intensifier (a large, portable, real-time X-ray machine) will be needed. If so, wheel it into the operating theatre, if the radiographer has not already done so.

The basic principles apply, of placing a tourniquet on the limb, and ensuring the limb is positioned to be manoeuvrable.

However, because the limb's skeletal support is broken, you will be required to take its place until it is repaired. This means providing traction – that is, maintaining the correct alignment of the fractured limb, usually by gently pulling along the long axis of the bone, to separate the ends of the fracture and prevent them from grinding together. Maintaining alignment of the limb ensures the neurovascular structures are not compromised – there is no point fixing a dead, avascular limb! You may need to continue maintaining traction to the fractured limb, whilst the surgeon preps and drapes the patient.

## ■ Preparation

Even in situations such as open fractures with severe contamination of the wound, sterility is still important. The aim of the surgery is to decontaminate the wound, and this is achieved by a combination of debridement of dead and devitalised tissue, and copious lavage. Therefore, standard sterility principles are observed during skin preparation and setting up of the equipment.

### Intra-operatively

You will need to continue to act as the body's replacement for the broken skeletal structure, maintaining the alignment of the limb as carefully as possible to avoid further neurovascular and soft tissue injury.

If a bone is to be internally fixed (either with a plate and screws or intramedullary nail) or externally fixed (external fixateur), you may need to hold the limb in position to assist with the reduction of the fracture. Sometimes this can be quite physically demanding. This can be a very intense and frustrating time for the surgeon. Be alert to the surgeon's every request for even the smallest of movements, and especially, remain motionless when requested to do so. It may seem like an eternity, but a minute of concentration can shorten the entire procedure. The surgeon will attempt to hold the reduction in place with clamps until definitive fixation with metal-work can be achieved. This is a critical time, and every effort should be made not to disturb the reduction until the fracture is definitively stabilised.

If intra-operative X-rays are performed, try to be constructive in assessing them. Do not try to coerce the surgeon into accepting a poor reduction or unacceptable screw placement, just to bring an end to a long and uncomfortable procedure. This helps no-one, particularly the patient.

## Post-operatively

As after elective surgery, you should check the distal blood supply, and collect all the X-rays and case-notes and place them on the patient's bed.

# ■ Tips for assisting at specific common operations

## Fractured neck of femur

### Subcapital fracture

If the fracture is undisplaced, the operation will very likely be an open reduction and internal fixation (ORIF)* as for a pertrochanteric fracture (see below). If it is displaced, then the surgeon will probably perform a hemiarthroplasty, that is, a partial joint replacement replacing the femoral side of the joint. In this case, the set-up and your role will be similar to that required for a total hip replacement.

### Pertrochanteric fracture

The standard operation is an ORIF. The patient will normally be placed on a traction table. You will have a very prominent role here, holding the limb as required, and supporting the surgeon as he or she straps the patient into the table. This is often the most labour-intensive part of this operation, and a good assistant helps prevent the surgeon becoming fatigued before the operation has even started.

The Image Intensifier is virtually always used for these cases, so ensure it is present before starting. During the operation, the position of the patient is usually such that there is only enough room for the surgeon to be close to the operative field, while you must stand further away. However, you may be called upon to retract tissues, so be alert.

## Distal radial fracture (Colles' fracture)

This common fracture is usually treated with a closed reduction, but your role is still very important. You will need to provide counter-traction on the upper forearm, while the surgeon puts traction on the hand and reduces the fracture. You must then maintain your position as still as possible, while the surgeon works vigorously to apply and mould the plaster before it sets.

---

* The pedantic may argue that, strictly, this is a closed reduction, as the fracture site is not directly exposed.

## 17

# Otorhinolaryngology- head and neck surgery

**Richard Douglas** MD, FRACS, FRACP, MRCP

Fellow, Department of Otolaryngology-Head and Neck Surgery

The Queen Elizabeth Hospital, Woodville, Australia

**Peter-John Wormald** MD, FRACS, FRCS, FCS(SA)

Professor, Department of Otolaryngology-Head and Neck Surgery

The Queen Elizabeth Hospital, Woodville, Australia

## ■ Introduction

Otorhinolaryngology-head and neck surgery (ORL-HNS) is a relatively new surgical subspecialty. It offers many challenges to the surgeon and his or her assistant because of the diversity of structures operated upon. These include the ear, nose, mouth, throat, larynx and neck. Thyroid and parathyroid surgery is being performed increasingly by head and neck surgeons, and facial plastic surgery is comprising a greater part of the ORL-HNS workload. Access to these structures is often limited and many of the structures are small, requiring either a microscope or endoscope to provide magnification for adequate visualization for surgery. Due to the proximity of vital structures, such as the brain, cranial nerves, eyes and large vascular structures, surgery can be very challenging and sometimes stressful. Some cases provide an extra challenge to both the anaesthetic and surgical teams by having compromised upper airways.

## ■ Preparation of the patient

As an assistant, it is always beneficial to your medical education, and often helpful to the smooth running of the surgical team, if you familiarise yourself with the patient's case-notes pre-operatively. Because of the complicated anatomy of the area, having the patient's CT or MRI scans available in the operating room is often important, and when possible you should review the scans on the light-box or computer screen preoperatively. For ear cases, locating the latest pure tone audiogram in the case-notes and knowing the extent of hearing deficit is advantageous. For all operations being performed on one side only, it is a potentially useful safeguard for you to know which is the correct side (see also p. 21).

Because the structures being operated on are frequently small and can be obscured by minimal haemorrhage, every attempt is made to reduce unnecessary bleeding. Most procedures are performed with the operating table tilted at 15–20° to horizontal (the anti-Trendelenburg position). This reduces tissue perfusion pressure to the head and neck, and encourages venous return. The anaesthetic team often induce hypotension during the operation for the same reason.

Skin preparation is generally performed with an aqueous povidone–iodine solution. It is important to ensure that alcohol based solutions are not used because these can injure the conjunctiva, and if they come into contact with the inner ear they have the potential to cause sensorineural deafness. Some common ORL-HNS procedures are performed under clean rather than sterile conditions: tonsillectomy and surgery inside the nose and sinuses are examples of procedures in which it is not possible to sterilise the operating field and so no attempt is made to do so. In the case of surgery on the throat and neck, the patient's oropharyngeal flora contaminates the surgical wound. Therefore, all patients undergoing ear, nose and major head and neck procedures are given prophylactic antibiotics.

Cases in which the upper airway is compromised always demand careful preoperative preparation and consultation between the surgical and anaesthetic teams, to ensure that back up plans are formulated to secure the compromised airway, and that any equipment needed to perform them is immediately available. If the airway is compromised by, for example, a laryngeal tumour then it is optimal to have a range of laryngoscopes available in the operating room (and particularly a Kleinsasser DL laryngoscope which can reach the subglottis, and through which a small endotracheal tube can be passed). A tracheotomy tray should be readily available. If there is significant concern about the establishment of a safe airway, then even before the anaesthetist begins to attempt intubation, the surgeon and yourself should be scrubbed and prepared to perform an emergency tracheotomy if needed.

## ■ Ear surgery

Most surgery on the middle and inner ear is performed with the aid of an operating microscope. Operating microscopes offer a stereoscopic view of the operating field and have hand controls which allow them to be moved easily over the field. Most have either a side viewing arm or alternatively a video system, which allow the assistant to follow the operation.

Ear operations are performed on very small and delicate structures. An extensive range of specialised instruments has been developed to facilitate the performance of operations on the ear. However, because of the limited surgical access, it is relatively uncommon for a surgeon who is performing ear procedures to require direct assistance.

## ■ Nasal surgery

Nasal surgery can be divided into procedures performed on the external nasal skeleton (septorhinoplasty) and those performed on internal structures (most commonly the septum, turbinates and paranasal sinuses).

Septorhinoplasty is a demanding procedure which is greatly facilitated by a skilled assistant. As with most surgical procedures, good exposure is the key to success and the assistant plays a vital role in retracting the nasal skin envelope with skin hooks or specialised retractors, such as an Aufricht retractor. The nasal tissues need to be handled delicately at all times. It is important that the plane between nasal cartilage and perichondrium is seen clearly, to speed dissection. You can gently remove blood from this plane with a cotton-tipped dressing probe. When osteotomies are being performed, you will usually help the surgeon by gently tapping the osteotome with a mallet.

Most surgery on the paranasal sinuses is performed transnasally with the aid of rigid endoscopes. Usually a video camera is fitted to the end of the endoscope, to enable the surgeon and his or her assistant to follow the procedure on a screen. As the endoscope has a diameter of 4 mm, generally only one more instrument can fit into the nostril. Therefore, most endoscopic sinus procedures are performed by the surgeon unassisted. However, in complicated procedures a small window can be cut in the nasal septum to allow access from the opposite nasal cavity. This allows the assistant to place a nasal sucker into the operating field to keep it free of blood while the surgeon continues to operate.

## ■ Head and neck surgery

The principles of assisting for head and neck procedures are similar to those of general surgical procedures. Tumour resections comprise the majority of the workload in most head and neck units. The procedures are often lengthy;

eight hours is not uncommon. This is both because of the anatomical demands of the region, and the need to reconstruct the surgical defect.

To restore form and function as much as possible, reconstruction of surgical defects is often done with flaps of skin, muscle and sometimes bone. These flaps are sometimes composed of nearby tissues which keep their own blood supply (and are therefore known as regional flaps). However, often the flap is composed of tissues from a remote part of the body. In this case, the blood vessels of the flap are divided and re-anastomosed with blood vessels in the head and neck (forming a free flap). Free flaps may be removed from parts of the body as distant as the fibula, and it is a good idea to revise the regional anatomy the night before assisting procedures outside your usual field of activity. It is common for two surgical teams to work simultaneously on major head and neck resections: while one team removes the tumour, the other raises the flap and then subsequently sutures it in place to cover the defect.

During surgery on the neck and larynx, the assistant is often required to retract delicate structures, such as skin flaps, and occasionally cranial nerves or important blood vessels, such as those which supply the brain. Rough handling of such structures can lead to significant functional deficits and in some cases may cause complications, with excessive traction rupturing delicate vessels compromised by tumour invasion. It is important to remain focussed on the task at hand, and handle the tissues as gently as possible. The usual format for this surgery is for the surgeon to elevate a skin flap exposing the larynx, trachea and underlying muscles and lymph nodes of the neck. Partial or total resection of the larynx may be required for tumour involving this organ. In addition, removal of all regional lymph nodes is required to remove cancer cells that may have drained into these lymph nodes from the tumour site. Assistants need to understand the anatomy of both the larynx and associated lymph nodes, and where the vital vascular and neural structures run in relation to these structures.

Gentle retraction of tissue with exposure of these structures will greatly facilitate the surgical dissection. Suction or swabbing of excess blood will also improve the surgical field and speed up the dissection. Follow the surgeon's instructions, but also try to anticipate the surgical steps, and provide retraction and swabbing that continuously gives the surgeon the clearest possible view of the region to be dissected.

# ■ Conclusions

Most surgical procedures on the ear and inside the nose do not require surgical assistance. Very gentle tissue handling for surgery on the external nose and during head and neck procedures can greatly facilitate the surgery and improve the surgical outcome for the patient.

## FURTHER READING

Bailey B (ed). *Atlas of Otolaryngology-Head and Neck Surgery.* Lippincott Williams and Wilkins, New York, USA 2002.
This large text has detailed descriptions and illustrations of the majority of ORL-HNS procedures.
Lee KJ (ed). *Essential Otolaryngology (8^{th} ed)*, Lange, Stamford, Connecticut USA 2003.
This single volume text book summarises the whole field of clinical ORL-HNS.

# Paediatric surgery

## 18

**Christopher Kirby** BMBS FRCS FRACS

Women's and Children's Hospital, North Adelaide, Adelaide, South Australia

When assisting at paediatric surgical operations, it is important to remember from the outset, that the differences between adults and children are not only in their size, anatomy and physiology, but also in their psychology. In particular, it is important not to frighten children in the operating theatre.

This is for at least two reasons. Firstly, just as in adult surgery, it is simply more pleasant for the patient (and parents and staff) if he or she is relaxed. Secondly, but unlike in adult surgery, a frightened infant or child patient greatly increases the difficulties faced by the anaesthetist. This is because a different method is commonly used for induction of anaesthesia ('going off to sleep') in this age group.

Whereas in adults the usual method for induction of anaesthesia is by intravenous injection, in children, the preferred method is more often by slow inhalation of anaesthetic gases. The main reason for using this method, is that it avoids the need to insert an intravenous cannula while the child is awake – an event that most children find distressing. Thus, intravenous induction can be something of a last resort in elective paediatric surgery, to be used when dealing with a child 'spooked' by the theatre environment.

The willing compliance of the child is required for gaseous induction. Therefore, prior to the induction of anaesthesia, it is particularly important to provide an atmosphere which is quiet, gentle and safe, enabling the parent and child to relax. Do not underestimate the value of frequent reassuring smiles. Try not to trivialise the parent's anxieties and concerns. In short, be friendly and professional.

## ■ Keep infants warm

All members of the surgical and anaesthetic team should be mindful of the needs of the unconscious patient. The needs of the child in the operating room vary with age, or more precisely, with weight. Neonates and infants under about 5 kg are acutely sensitive to cooling due to their very low body weight in proportion to their surface area. In neonates, and less commonly in larger infants and toddlers, hypothermia can have serious consequences, such as hypoglycaemia and apnoea.

Hypothermia can occur in such patients even during short procedures, if specific measures to prevent it are not taken. These measures include pre-warming the operating room, and ensuring the on-table heating blanket is properly connected. While adult operating rooms are typically maintained at about 21°C, neonatal operating rooms are markedly warmer: usually about 26°C.

Becoming wet during the procedure puts the infant at risk of more rapid chilling, and is commonly caused by the baby lying on drapes soaked by skin preparation solution.

## ■ Positioning child, airway and lines

The smaller the patient, the closer the airway (and for that matter all other parts of the patient) to the operative site. Surgeons and assisting surgeons need to be mindful of the exact position of the child under the drapes. Dislodging the laryngeal mask with an inadvertent surgical elbow, or bruising an infant's knee with a resting surgical fore-arm, are potentially serious events. Similarly, the intravenous access site is at risk of dislodgment, particularly at the conclusion of the procedure when drapes are being withdrawn. This entirely preventable event is irritating during any operation, but particularly so in paediatric surgery. This is because insertion of intravenous cannulae is distressing to small children, and is often technically difficult (due to their small veins in plump, mobile limbs).

## ■ Skin preparation

The antiseptic solution should be pre-warmed in the blanket warmer or other incubator and decanted into the 'prep set' immediately prior to use. Care should be taken to avoid spilling prep fluid in puddles around the infant or between the infant and the diathermy return plate.

## ■ Local anaesthetic considerations

Like all other drugs, the dosing and administration of local anaesthetic (LA) agents in children is calculated on a per weight basis. It is customary to confirm the intended dose with the anaesthetist before injecting LA. This is because at times, the anaesthetist may have administered an ilio-inguinal or caudal LA block in the induction room prior to surgery, thus significantly limiting the further administration of LA that could be safely given by wound infiltration at the conclusion of surgery.

# ■ Retraction

Expert retraction by the surgical assistant is fundamental to most non-laparoscopic procedures in children. Self-retaining retractors are rarely used in paediatric surgery, as their use requires a larger wound area relative to the small patient, and the retractor teeth tend to be unforgiving on infant tissue. Paired, small hand held retractors are far superior in the right hands for nearly all paediatric head and neck, abdominal and groin procedures (see also p. 71).

As in other areas of surgery, knowledge of the steps of the procedure being undertaken will greatly enhance your ability to assist, because you will be able to anticipate what is coming next and in which direction the surgeon will need the wound to be retracted. Surgeons are generally creatures of habit and tend to perform the same procedure in the same stepwise order every time. The second and subsequent inguinal herniotomy will therefore be significantly easier for you than the first.

# ■ Specific regions

## Thoracotomy

The chest of the infant is short relative to the adult, and the incompletely ossified ribs compliant. Therefore lateral or postero-lateral fifth space thoracotomy in the lateral decubitus position provides satisfactory access for most oesophageal and lung surgery, without the need for rib division or resection. However, before pubertal growth, the major airways are relatively narrow and thus lung isolation by way of a dual-lumen endotracheal tube more difficult. Consequently, it is common for paediatric thoracic operations to be done with both lungs inflated. It follows that, as an assistant, you may often find that you are required to retract (and therefore, usually compress) the lung enough for the surgeon's access, but are limited by the needs of the anaesthetist for adequate ventilation.

The infant's tissues are delicate, and especially so in the chest. Therefore, it is extremely important that you handle the tissues with great care and gentleness. For example, the infant lung is easily lacerated when handled with forceps or vigorous direct suction. The pulmonary veins are the thinnest-walled large vessels in humans, and in young children cannot be grasped safely, even with vascular clamps. Therefore, to minimise the chance of injury to these structures, all instruments enter the infant chest in the surgeon's hand and are then transferred to you, the assistant, as required.

## Laparotomy

Children have a short, relatively wide abdomen with the umbilicus significantly closer to the pubis than xiphisternum. The pelvis is shallow, with the bladder very much an abdominal rather then deep pelvic organ in the first years of life. For all these reasons, open access to the abdominal cavity is most commonly via a transverse incision (e.g. for pyloromyotomy, fundoplication, or intussusception). Therefore, when you assist at a paediatric laparotomy, your hand will be retracting up over the infant's chest or head and you must be mindful of leaning on the patient or displacing the endotracheal tube.

## The groin

Possibly due to the complexity of complete genital development in the human male, the surgical correction of hernias, hydroceles, undescended testes and the penis comprises the vast majority of general paediatric day surgery. Largely to protect the toddler and school age child from the psychological traumas of hospital admission, anaesthesia and genital surgery, these procedures are now commonly performed during the first 2 years. The surgical target is thus small and the surgeon will often use surgical magnifying glasses (loupes). Wearing these instruments significantly restricts the surgeon's field of vision, so he will be relying on you and the scrub nurse to provide everything within his limited (even though magnified) visual field.

## Indwelling catheters

After an operation, if you are left to secure a urinary catheter or other drain, be mindful of the numerous ways in which these can be removed; sometimes deliberately by children, usually accidentally by their carers. Catheters are best strapped to the lower abdomen or groin crease, but never the thigh. This is because, when the child jumps or sits cross-legged, the thigh moves laterally, pulling the catheter (and its balloon!) through the urethra, or perhaps even worse, through the urethral repair.

To keep the patient's hands off the catheter, use double nappies, or tape the top of the nappy to the skin. Do not tape the catheter to the bag tubing. If mother picks up the child and walks away from the cot, it is much better for the catheter tube to come apart at this junction rather than pull the whole device from the patient.

### SUGGESTED FURTHER READING

Keith W Ashcraft (ed) *et al.* Pediatric Surgery (4th edition), Elsevier Saunders. London, 2005.

# Plastic surgery and microsurgery

19

**Graham J Offer** BSc(Hons) MBChB FRCS(Eng) FRCS(Plast)

Leicester Royal Infirmary, Leicester, England

## ■ Introduction

Plastic surgeons perform many types of procedures to correct deformities and reconstruct tissue defects. The specialty covers all age groups and body areas. Consequently, you may encounter plastic surgeons working with most other specialties, at some point or other. If you are assisting at small cases you may be the only assistant, whereas in large cases there may be two or three surgeons and two scrub teams (see p. 2). One thing that is common to all plastic surgeons is that they are sticklers for good technique. Therefore, you should show care in handling all body tissues.

## ■ Plastic surgical terms

### Graft

This is a piece of tissue (usually skin) that is detached from one area of the body (the donor site) and then placed on another area, such as a wound (the bed). At the end of the procedure it does not have a blood supply, but will acquire this from the bed over the next few days, rather like rolls of bare-rooted turf taking root in the underlying soil. The process of gaining this blood supply is termed 'graft take'. Obviously therefore, a graft can only be used on a bed that has an adequate blood supply. For example, a graft cannot be used to cover a wound with a large metal plate in the centre of the bed (just as a roll of turf will not survive on bare rock).

### Flap

This is a piece of tissue (skin, muscle, bone or viscera) that is moved from one area of the body to another, but which continues to receive its blood supply from the normal blood vessels it contains. These vessels are termed 'the pedicle'.

If the supplying blood vessels are left intact, then it is called a 'pedicled flap' and it can only be moved as far as the vessels will physically allow. However, if the supplying vessels are divided and then joined to other vessels elsewhere (using microsurgery), then it is called a 'free flap'. A free flap can be moved to any area of the body as long as its blood vessels can be joined onto the vessels of that region.

Consequently, unlike grafts, both pedicled and free flaps can be used to cover any bed, because their blood supply is not dependent upon the bed.

## ■ Instruments in plastic surgery

Plastic surgeons tend to use fine operating instruments, such as Adson's or Gillies toothed forceps (see Figures 10.12 and 10.13).

When the surgeon has many small sutures to place, (such as when operating on complex facial wounds), he or she will often use a specialised plastic surgical needle-holder, such as a Gillies or a Foster. These instruments differ from ordinary needle-holders in that they are something of a hybrid between a needle-holder and a pair of scissors. That is, they have no ratchet, and have scissor blades on their shafts. Thus, they allow the surgeon to save time by both inserting sutures and then trimming them, using only one instrument. Fine ratcheted needle-holders (such as Kilner or Nieverts) are also used frequently. These are sometimes palm held.

As an assistant, you will commonly be asked to provide gentle retraction of the skin. Instruments you will use for this include skin hooks for finer work, and the Kilner (cats paw) retractor for heavier skin (see Figure 10.18).

When you are assisting a surgeon raising a large composite tissue flap, you will often use one of the general surgical retractors (such as the Czerny, Deaver or Langenbeck). Use traction and counter-traction to separate tissue planes (see pp. 51–3). Headlights and lighted retractors are sometimes used if operating down a hole.

Endoscopic equipment may occasionally be used for raising flaps (see Chapter 12, p. 103).

Some surgeons have preferences for particular glove types, for procedures such as microsurgery.

### Cutting sutures (see also p. 57)

Cut sutures short enough that the trimmed end will not catch in the next suture, but long enough that the sutures are easy to remove, and not at risk of the knot unravelling (see Figure 10.5). For interrupted skin sutures, this is usually about 3 mm length. If in doubt, ask the surgeon.

Sometimes, a surgeon will place deep dermal sutures when closing a wound. In this case, he or she may ask you to trim the suture right down at skin level, so as not to leave any suture ends protruding from the wound.

# ■ Assisting at skin grafting procedures

## Split thickness grafts

These contain the epidermis and a variable thickness of the dermis. The donor site will heal by regrowth of the epidermis from epidermal cells that are located within the hair follicles and sweat glands.

The commonest donor site for a split skin graft is the thigh. Therefore, the following description assumes the thigh is the donor site, but the general principles of assisting apply to any site.

The surgeon will use a skin graft knife (e.g. Watson, Humby or Braithwaite) or a mechanical dermatome (such as a Zimmer, usually for larger graft harvests, e.g. burns cases). The surgeon will set the graft knife or dermatome to the desired thickness of cut. Some liquid paraffin or saline may be applied to the skin to lubricate the blade as it cuts. You may do this while the surgeon adjusts the knife.

The surgeon will then pass the blade along the skin of the thigh, with the blade cutting a thin layer of skin as it goes, rather like a cheese-slicer or a carpenter's plane. To give a graft of even thickness, the skin needs to present a flat surface to the blade and to be kept taught under tension. As the assistant, you will play an important part in providing this skin presentation.

Do this by pulling the skin taught around the thigh, by placing your hands on the opposite side of the thigh to the intended donor site, and grasping the skin and soft tissues firmly (see Figure 19.1). This is sometimes called the 'donkey-bite' manoeuvre. At the same time, push the tissue towards the knife to present a flat surface to the blade, rather than a cylindrical one. Some surgeons may also press a flat wooden board against the skin, to stretch out the skin and flatten it as they cut.

Once cut, a split skin graft may be meshed before application to the bed. This means that it is placed upon a board and passed through a small machine (that looks a bit like a mangle) which puts perforations in the graft. The graft then looks a bit like a string vest. The perforations allow the graft to be expanded to one and a half, three or six times its size, dependent upon the distance between the perforations. The other purpose of meshing is to permit blood and tissue fluid that forms beneath the graft, to seep out through the perforations and so not interfere with the graft 'take'.

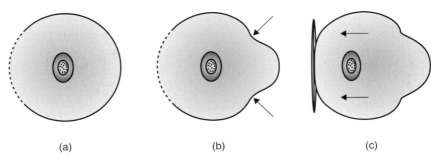

(a)                          (b)                          (c)

**Figure 19.1**  This shows a cross-section of the thigh during harvest of a split-thickness skin graft. (a) The thigh, with the site of the intended skin graft indicated by the dotted line. (b) The assistant firmly grasps the skin and soft tissues of the thigh as indicated by the arrows; this 'donkey-bite manoeuvre' tenses the skin at the graft site. (c) While maintaining skin tension with the 'donkey-bite', the assistant pushes the tissues towards the graft site as indicated by the arrows. This helps to present a flat surface to the graft knife. In the illustration, the surgeon is also pressing a board against the skin as a further aid to presenting a flat surface.

It is vital to place the graft 'shiny side down' (cut surface down) otherwise it will not 'take'.

### Full thickness grafts

These contain the epidermis and all of the dermis. Because all the skin elements are removed, the donor site will not heal and is usually directly closed by suturing the skin edges together.

Both full-thickness and split-thickness grafts should be kept moist with saline soaked gauze until required, and not allowed to dry out.

## ■ Assisting at flap procedures

### Pedicled flaps

Obviously, survival of a flap depends on an intact blood supply, so it is crucial not to damage the pedicle. Therefore, take care when holding the flap or retracting it. Do not pull on the pedicle, or you may accidentally damage it or even avulse it. When cutting sutures, use the tips of the scissors so that you do not accidentally cut the pedicle (see Figure 10.3).

When the flap is raised, be careful if using monopolar diathermy on it, as the current will flow down the pedicle and could damage it. Instead of lifting the flap away from the body, press the flap down against the body so that the current does not flow down the pedicle.

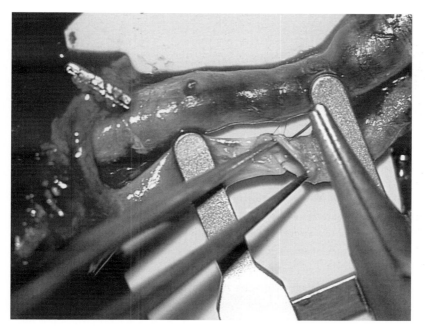

**Figure 19.2** End-to-end microvascular venous anastomosis with 10/0 ethilon suture. The vessels have been placed in a microvascular double clamp.

## Free flaps

The principles of assisting are similar to those for pedicled flaps, but there is also the microsurgery to assist with (see below).

# ■ Microsurgery

This is a highly specialised area of surgery and you are unlikely to be assisting at this type of surgery on an *ad hoc* basis. Nevertheless, here are some tips for you if you are new to the area or are unexpectedly called upon to help.

By far the commonest microsurgical operations are anastomoses of blood vessels, and it is therefore suggested that readers also refer to the chapter on assisting at vascular surgery (Chapter 22, p. 172). Obviously, in microvascular surgery, the blood vessels that are anastomosed are very small: usually in the order of 1–3 mm in diameter (see Figure 19.2). Specialised sutures and instruments are therefore needed, as is magnification, usually in the form of an operating microscope.

The surgeon may anastomose the vessels end-to-end as shown in the photograph. Alternatively, vessels may be anastomosed end-to-side (e.g. when the vessels are of different diameters ('size mismatch') and will not join easily, end-to-end).

## Equipment

### Microscope

The microscope is usually set up before it is needed. To allow the surgeon to adjust it intra-operatively, it may be draped with a sterile cover, or sterile handles may be put on the controls. Most microscopes have two sets of eyepieces: one for the surgeon and one directly opposite for the assistant. Some microscopes have the assistant eyepiece on a side arm or have this side arm in addition for teaching purposes.

The first step should be to set up your microscope eyepieces. Comfort is imperative. In particular, you should not be bending your neck uncomfortably. If you wear spectacles, the eyepieces may be set to your own prescription, or you may set them to zero and wear your spectacles.

The microscope is wheeled into position. The surgeon will move the lens system to lie above the area of the anastomosis. With older microscopes, knobs are then tightened to fix all of the joints solidly in position. Newer microscopes have handles much like a submarine periscope, with a button to press which automatically fixes all of the joints solid. The surgeon will focus the microscope, and you should then find that your view is also in focus. If not, then you will need to adjust your eyepieces.

Once the operation is underway, try not to move your eyes away from the microscope view. Ask for instruments and hold out your hand to the theatre nurse (or operating department practitioner), who will take the instrument in your hand and replace it with the requested one.

### Sutures

Unsurprisingly, the sutures used in microsurgery are very fine and delicate: usually 9/0 or 10/0. They are often finer than a human hair (Figure 19.3).

### Commonly used microvascular instruments

Refer to Figure 19.4.

### How to hold microsurgery instruments (Figures 19.5 and 19.6)

Steadiness and comfort are paramount. Some surgeons put rolled up towels under their fore-arms, or use special seats which have arm supports attached. Microsurgery movements are mainly at finger-joint level, rather than at the fore-arm. The ulnar border of the hand is steadied against the patient or operating

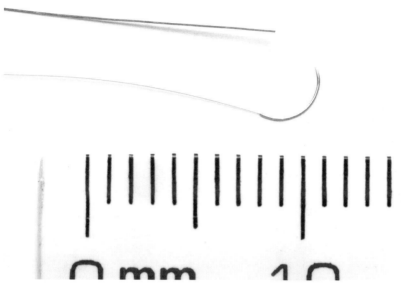

**Figure 19.3** 10/0 microsurgical needle with suture next to a human hair.

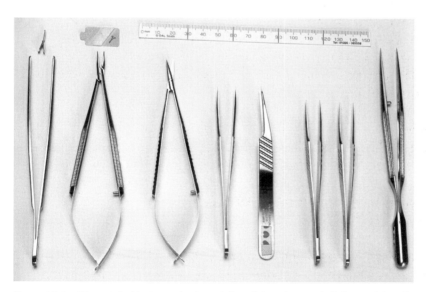

**Figure 19.4** Microsurgical instruments. From left to right: microsurgical clamp and applicator; needle-holder (with needle in 'parking bay'); straight microscissors; pair of vessel dilators; pair of short handled jeweller's forceps size 5; long handled jeweller's forceps.

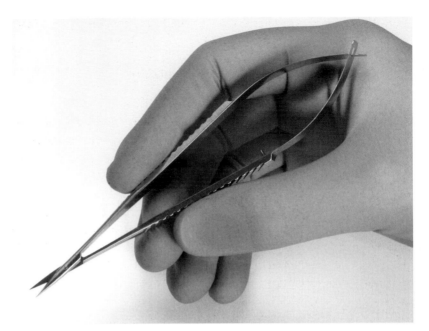

Figure 19.5   Holding microsurgical scissors 'open'.

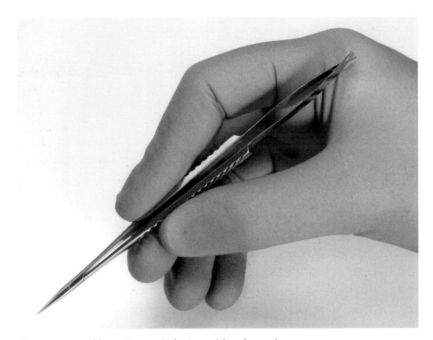

Figure 19.6   Holding microsurgical scissors 'closed to cut'.

table to steady the tripod of thumb, index and middle finger. Some advocate caffeine avoidance to help prevent tremor, but this is fairly subjective.

## Quiet during microsurgery (see also, 'talking in the operating theatre', p. 6)

To minimise the time a flap is ischaemic, the surgeon will aim to minimise the time between removal of the flap from the body ('flap off') and the time of completion of the microsurgery, and consequent restoration of blood flow to the flap ('flap on'). The time from 'flap off' to 'flap on' should be recorded.

Intense concentration is therefore required, since one wrongly placed stitch may cause a vascular thrombosis with consequent failure of the entire procedure. No loud conversations amongst staff members in theatre should take place during the microsurgery. Surgeons have been known to become very displeased with theatre staff who talk loudly about their social lives, whilst the surgeon is trying to perform this technically challenging procedure.

The author and many other surgeons enjoy music while they are operating. However, during the microsurgical part of the procedure, the author finds it more appropriate either to turn off the sound system completely or to listen to relaxing music (so turn from Meatloaf to Mozart).

## Handling tissues

The blood vessels of the pedicle are very delicate. This is especially so of the inner layer of the vessels (the intima). Injury to this layer can easily lead to thrombosis and flap failure. Therefore, handle the vessels with great care, and avoid touching the intima unnecessarily.

Take great care when wielding the sucker. Especially, do not plunge it into the vessel lumen and suck on the intima. Some surgeons advocate sucking on a small patty which is placed in the wound (see also, 'neurosurgery', p. 120). If using spears (triangular patties on sticks), dab gently with them when asked. Use a syringe of heparinised saline for irrigation (or 'hydroflow' system).

Never grab the ends of the vessels with the forceps. Instead, gently handle the vessels by their outer layer (the adventitia).

To allow positioning of a suture in an awkward site, the surgeon may ask you to hold up stay sutures with jeweller's forceps.

When you are cutting sutures, the surgeon should let you know how long the suture ends should be. Do not get your scissors in the surgeon's way. Move your instruments into the operating field, only when the surgeon asks (e.g. when asked to cut the suture). This way you will not knock the surgeon's instruments.

If you need to pass the needle to the surgeon, let him or her take it under magnification from the 'parking bay' (a needle-storing device, see Figure 19.4).

Some surgeons use hand signals to ask the scrub nurse for particular instruments. Therefore, don't be surprised when you see the surgeon suddenly using a new instrument down the microscope, when you didn't even hear him or her ask for one.

## Assisting when the microscope has no assistant's eyepiece

Some theatres may only have a microscope with one eyepiece. In this case, sometimes a video camera feed of the microscope view can be displayed on a screen, to allow you to assist. Otherwise, you will either need to look carefully with the naked eye, wear operating loupes or simply tell the surgeon that you cannot see the sutures to cut them, and 'bail out' of assisting.

## Dressings

Most plastic surgeons will want to put the dressings on the wounds themselves, and consider this part of their surgical role. Particular attention should be paid to the dressings, since a shoddily applied dressing may lead the patient to believe that the same care was used for the surgery!

It is vital that the dressings do not restrict the blood flow to or from a flap. Plastic surgeons are very particular to ensure that the procedure does not fail due to venous congestion caused by tight dressings.

When reconstructing the head and neck region with microvascular free flaps, the same rule applies to tapes used to secure a tracheostomy tube in place. These tapes can constrict the flow of blood through the pedicle, leading to flap failure. Consequently, the surgeon may elect to suture the tracheostomy tube to the skin, rather than use the tapes.

## Conclusion

Good assistance comes with teamwork. You are likely to improve if you get a dedicated job in the microsurgery theatres. In the meantime, you could try and learn telepathy.

# Surgery in difficult circumstances: (1) Rural hospitals

## 20

**Martin Bruening** BMBS MS FRCS(Ed) FRACS

The Queen Elizabeth Hospital, Woodville, Adelaide, South Australia
Port Augusta Hospital, Port Augusta, South Australia

Many rural towns are not big enough to need a full-time resident surgeon, but instead rely on visiting surgeons to provide the necessary expertise for elective cases. Often, the surgeons only stay overnight, and are then on the move again. This arrangement is very common in Australia, due to its sheer size and the widespread distribution of its towns.

In this situation, it is predominantly the general practitioner (GP) who acts as the surgical assistant. In larger towns, the surgical assisting duties may fall to a GP who has a designated interest in surgery, or the duties may be assigned via a roster system. However in many cases, the referring GP will be the surgical assistant. With the current trend of increasing medical undergraduate exposure to the rural environment, most regional centres will have medical students available to act as surgical assistants. While many of the concepts of assisting have been covered elsewhere in the text, there are several points which should be highlighted.

## ■ Tips for the GP

If you are new to a particular region or town, introduce yourself to the operating theatre staff. This helps to break the ice and ensure that you are on a good footing with the nursing staff. When introducing yourself to the surgeon, always call them by their correct title to begin with, and then let them tell you, 'Please call me Bob', etc.

Punctuality is of the essence as the visiting surgeon is often on a tight schedule, and will not appreciate being kept waiting. Obviously, if you are attending an emergency situation no-one will quibble, but a phone call through to theatre may enable cases to be reorganised and the list can continue.

Keep an open mind when dealing with surgeons for the first time. It is amazing how many times a surgeon's reputation for being 'difficult' in the city seems completely at odds with their behaviour in the country setting. Most surgeons enjoy providing a service to the rural community and the 'country run' is a highlight in their surgical practice.

Do not assume that all surgeons operate with the same technique. While there is a framework of standard steps for every surgical procedure, there are many subtle variations along the way. There is nothing more frustrating for a surgeon to be told for the umpteenth time that, 'Mr Neil never does this'.

As the doctor providing on-going care for the patient, it is important to ask the surgeon about post-operative orders, follow-up and potential problems and how to recognise them. The best time to ask about these things is during changeover between cases. The most important question to ask is 'How can I contact you in the event that there is a problem?'

## ■ Tips for the medical student

Most surgeons will be delighted with having medical students as assistants, as this gives them an opportunity to teach in a way which is increasingly less possible in the tertiary metropolitan hospital setting. Introduce yourself to the surgeon and ask if it is permissible for you to assist. If there is more than one student available to scrub, it is always worth asking whether an additional assistant is needed. If you are not sure what the surgeon is asking you to do while assisting, always ask.

One of the golden rules for medical students is to never get the scrub sister offside.

This can be avoided by the following simple instructions:

1  Always introduce yourself to the scrub sister prior to the procedure.
2  Listen to what the scrub sister has to say.
3  Never grab anything from the instrument tray.
4  Laugh at the sister's jokes.

The second golden rule for assisting students is that if you find yourself feeling light headed, and hear yourself utter the words, 'Is it me , or is everyone hot in here ?', you must step back from the operating table and sit down on the floor as you have 9.46 seconds until you faint. There is absolutely no disgrace or embarrassment in adopting this approach and if the truth be known, most individuals who work within the confines of the operating theatre have experienced this phenomenon early in their careers.

Most of the suggestions for GP assisting apply equally to medical students, although it is not advisable for students to address surgeons by their Christian names, unless invited to do so.

# Surgery in difficult circumstances: (2) Developing countries

21

**Peter Riddell** FRACS

Flinders Medical Centre, Bedford Park, Adelaide, South Australia and Visiting Surgeon, various rural hospitals in South-East Asia

Surgical work in the developing world can be one of the most rewarding experiences in a surgical career. You are an essential component of an essential team, in an area where medical resources are scarce or minimal. Almost without exception, your contribution will be highly valued. You will be making a difference. The experience can also be very frustrating. Frustrating, because you will generally be operating under less than ideal circumstances, and will not always be able to achieve what is possible in the developed world.

This chapter is written primarily for assistants who normally work in the developed world, and plan to work in a developing country either on a short- or long-term basis. It describes the overall nature of surgery and assisting in such circumstances, rather than on techniques for assisting at individual procedures.

Points for consideration have been divided into those of a general nature and those more specific to assisting.

## ■ General considerations

### Standards

For those of us who work primarily in the developed world, perhaps the most difficult concept to accept is that standards of care in developing countries will differ from those we are used to 'at home'. For example, surgical sterility is very hard to achieve in any developing world setting. There are several reasons for this. Theatre linen will probably be old and in short supply. The linen may not be correctly washed between cases to the standards to which we are accustomed. Sterilisation techniques may not render it completely sterile; sterilisers are expensive to run and maintain, and replacement parts may not be available. The pressure of work, and humid conditions in tropical climates, may mandate the use of damp linen – another reason for non-sterility. Therefore, in developing countries, most surgical operations are surgically clean, rather than sterile.

Similarly, different standards will be in use both within the operating theatre (in terms of facilities and equipment) and also in patient care, pre-operatively, intra-operatively and post-operatively. There may be no auditing of surgical procedures and results. Consequently there is great potential for slipping of surgical standards, for not examining surgical outcomes and not instituting improved practices and procedures.

It is very easy to be critical of such a situation. The temptation is to make comparisons with the developed world ('we do it this way in our hospital') and so try to import or insist upon standards which are unachievable on a long-term basis. Generally there is a reason for the standards adopted. Perhaps they are dictated by cost, or by a lack of knowledge.

As a surgical assistant, you must accept that the challenge is firstly to understand and work within these differing conditions, *and then* aim to change the standards. There is no place for criticism without a practical solution.

References to surgical standards (made or implied) further in the text are given on the understanding that they are not meant as criticism, but rather as statements of fact.

## Cultural matters

### Language

It is challenging to work in any culture different to one's own. It is made much easier by being able to speak the local language. Obviously, working in an English-speaking country will usually make it even easier, but misunderstandings are still possible; words, phrases, intonation or gestures may be interpreted differently by local and western speakers. There will also be an eagerness on both sides not to 'lose face', and culturally it may not be appropriate to admit that either party cannot understand the meaning of the other. This especially applies to those for whom English is a second language. Hence, there may be apparent understanding of what is being said, but in reality, little true comprehension.

Working in a non-English-speaking country is even more difficult and may require an interpreter, unless one is fluent in the language. Still, if you maintain a friendly and smiling attitude, it is surprising how much understanding there can be with very little language skills.

On no account should you lose your temper, or display signs of annoyance or frustration. (Of course, this is easier said than done.) In many cultures, these emotions are signs of human failings or weakness, and you will be viewed accordingly thereafter. It is difficult to redeem such a situation. You may well find yourself tolerated, but excluded from further activities.

The author experienced just such a testing incident, when a valuable reusable (and non-replaceable) piece of surgical equipment was thrown out and incinerated at the end of an operation. It was said to be 'lost', despite the author having previously explained to local staff that the item should be looked after carefully, with apparent understanding on their part ('yes' many times). One's natural instinct at the time is to become angry, dwell on the subject and point out to everyone how other patients will be disadvantaged by the loss, through cancellation of operations. This approach is likely to be a loser for all concerned. The equipment cannot be recovered, so you personally will not be satisfied. The local staff member who lost the equipment may be dismissed, so losing an income which may be supporting more than one family. It will likely have an effect on other staff. Their relationship to you may mean that you have poor co-operation thereafter: either because they do not respect you or because they are scared to upset you, and find that avoiding tasks will prevent them getting into trouble. They may consider this to be better than the risk of being humiliated in front of others should you lose your temper.

The best solution is to accept the loss, point out that it has occurred and accept responsibility – say that it was your fault (which may have been a factor) for not adequately explaining the importance of the equipment to those concerned. You will find that it never happens again: those responsible will have learned by their mistake, there is 'no loss of face' and you gain, rather than lose, respect from the local people.

## Work productivity

Work productivity and ethics may be very different to those which you experience in the western world. The reasons are likely to be multifactorial, and complex. Local staff income, education, motivation to work, differing values on life, social status of the patients and money available for surgical procedures are some of the reasons. You should be aware of these, work within the constraints and try to make changes when appropriate. Applying high and consistent standards will be the best way of earning respect and making future changes.

An example is a patient requiring an urgent life-saving operation, and an inability to find staff to open the operating theatre. Eventually the theatre is activated either later that day or the next (after apparently more important home, family or political matters). The patient subsequently dies. This outcome may be explained to you as being inevitable ('never seen one survive before'). It is made more difficult since in the western world, you may have seen many similar cases, helped to treat them and seen them survive. You know that there is a high likelihood that the patient would have survived even in the current circumstances, if you had been able to get him or her to the theatre earlier.

This situation may be difficult to rationalise. Again, you need to accept that it has happened and that it is counterproductive in the first instance to show annoyance and lay blame, especially without knowing all the facts. The challenge is to change practices and let people see that such cases can survive. It must be remembered that local staff will almost certainly not have the education, experience and depth of knowledge which you have been fortunate enough to attain. Teaching about the condition and the reasons and need for urgent surgery, will go a long way towards instituting change.

## The surgical team

Many assistants working in the developing world will be members of a visiting overseas surgical team. This should be a true 'team' experience, in which each member contributes within his or her area of expertise. It is a very good way to be introduced to developing world surgery. A team offers advantages in problem solving, in using multiple and varied resources, and in personal and team debriefing. However, you must be aware that a team of westerners is likely to stay together and to speak only English, and hence miss out on the integration with the local people which a smaller group will experience. You should try as much as possible to speak in the local language and interact with, and learn from, the local staff. You will be richer for it.

You should also remember that working with a team of people in a foreign environment can be stressful. You will probably be living, working and socialising together. It is likely that there will be disagreements between team members, which can however be resolved by compromise, patience and setting realistic goals.

If you are working in the developing world as a lone individual with local staff, you will quickly become integrated into the team. You will almost certainly find that many aspects of the surgery are different from those you have seen in the developed world. You may find that, because of your western experience, you are consulted on conditions and in situations which are beyond your knowledge. It is best to acknowledge that you do not know the answers being sought, rather than pretend you do.

## Personal safety

Working in the developing world is likely to be more hazardous than in your own country. However, these risks can be minimised. Your greatest risks are trauma from motor vehicle accidents, and infectious diseases.

### Trauma

Most developing countries have poor roads that lack safety features. Vehicles will probably be old and poorly maintained, without seatbelts, or even if seatbelts are present, the people will rarely wear them. A saving grace is that many roads are in such a condition that they do not allow fast speeds. Road travel needs planning accordingly.

### Infectious diseases

Infectious disease are common, with most being gastrointestinal. You should heed the usual precautions of enquiring about the safety of drinking water (and using bottled water if in doubt), avoiding ice, and only eating at food outlets recommended by local staff. If you become sick, not only will this be unpleasant for you, but also, you will be of no use to your patients. Furthermore, if you are part of a team, your illness may markedly reduce the benefit of the team, because other team members may need to care for you.

Many countries have endemic malaria and other mosquito-borne diseases. Most westerners have little immunity to these diseases. You will need to take appropriate prophylaxis. Hence you should seek medical travel advice well before leaving, to ensure you have all the appropriate immunisations.

### Fatigue

Fatigue may be a problem when working in an overseas environment. It has a variety of causes. You will probably be working long hours. You may have difficulty in getting to sleep, because your sleeping quarters are hot, humid and unfamiliar, and you are thinking about patients you have treated. Once asleep, you may be awoken by unfamiliar noises, including that rooster outside the window who must have over-the-horizon radar, anticipating sunrise. Fatigue will markedly impair your work, and should be avoided through anticipation. You may need to resort to using ear-plugs or relaxation techniques.

### Hydration

Particularly in tropical climates, it is easy to become dehydrated without realising it, even when in the operating theatre. Again, prevention is best. Consciously monitor your urine colour and daily urinary output (through urinary frequency), to encourage yourself to keep drinking water, in what may appear initially to be overly large amounts.

# ■ Specific considerations for surgical assisting

## Operating theatre conditions

The operating theatre is likely to differ to that in which you normally work. The theatre itself may be smaller than that to which you are accustomed. Theatre temperature control may be non-existent or inappropriate. The patient may be either too hot or too cold; the latter being more common, especially when air-conditioners are used. There may not be continuous suction (intermittent suction machine) or wall-piped oxygen (oxygen may be delivered in cylinders or via an oxygen concentrator). The electricity and water supplies may be intermittent. Even when functioning normally, the theatre lights may give less than expected illumination or inappropriate heating during use. Use of a battery-powered head torch is therefore highly recommended, particularly for operations which occur at night.

Diathermy is likely to be monopolar only (no bipolar). The theatre table will almost certainly be manually operated, and may not have been regularly serviced. The usual ancillary equipment for patient positioning may be difficult to locate.

Flies and other insects may be able to enter the operating theatre. Theatre cleaning protocols and standards may differ from those in the developed world.

## Specific operating theatre safety

Safety standards in the operating theatre are likely to be lower than those in the developed world:

1 The infectious status of the patient may not be adequately known. In many places tuberculosis (TB) is common. It may present as a pulmonary infection (with the patient coughing, potentially producing aerosol droplet spread), as a cold abscess (e.g. destroyed neck nodes which require surgical drainage, with spread of infectious pus), or with joint or bone surgical presentations. Obviously

the material is infective, and TB may be transmitted to you if you are unaware of the diagnosis and do not take adequate precautions.

Similarly, the HIV and hepatitis status of the patient may well not be known. Accordingly, you should treat all patients with Universal Precautions.

Blood transfusion screening may be similarly inadequate. This has implications in disease transmission (e.g. when the patient's relatives are the blood donors). You should be very careful if you personally have an open wound, and avoid surgical scrubbing and assisting.

Eye protection is essential, for all the reasons outlined above.

2 The surgical instruments may not be as sharp or of the quality of those in the developed world. Surgical scalpel blades become blunt quickly. Paradoxically, these are more dangerous than sharp ones. More force is required to cut, so that if the blade slips, it does so with more force and less control. Blunt surgical needles have similar properties. Instrument handling should be appropriately careful to avoid needle-stick injuries or worse.

3 Theatre gowns or gloves may not be impervious to contaminated patient blood or secretions. The gloves may be in short supply and have to be reused.

4 Theatre footwear may be minimal, such as simple open shoes like 'flip-flops' ('thongs') or sandals. These provide almost no protection in case of accidental dropping of instruments. It is worth considering bringing suitable theatre footwear with you when working in the developing world.

5 As outlined above, insects can be expected to get into the operating theatre. These insects may include mosquitoes, and as you stand assisting at the operating table, you are a stationary target unable to swipe at your assailants. You can therefore catch mosquito-borne diseases, such as malaria or dengue fever whilst assisting. Consequently, apply adequate skin protection pre-operatively, as well as taking the other prophylactic measures alluded to earlier.

6 You may be working with a surgeon trained in different surgical techniques from those to which you are accustomed. Hence the surgeon may not be able to anticipate your actions and vice versa. Appropriate care needs to be taken to avoid sharps injury.

7 Electrical equipment may be incorrectly wired, or it may have different earthing and connection systems from those with which you are familiar.

## Instruments

Instruments may be in short supply, old and/or worn. Many will have been donated through overseas aid. Unfortunately, often such instruments are donated because they are outdated and no longer required by the donor country. Hence, you will be working in an already difficult environment with instruments which may be substandard. You will soon learn why local surgeons view foreign aid with some scepticism. Improvisation is commonly required.

The normal swaged surgical sutures used in the western world may be too expensive for everyday use in developing countries. Instead, spooled suture material and reusable needles may be used. You should be familiar with the technique of threading the needle. The suture material will be on a spool, in a tube of preservative with a bung top through which the end of the thread protrudes (see Figure 21.1). When a suture is required, the theatre nurse will draw out the appropriate length of thread, cut off the unsterile end and thread the needle, generally using a single-handed technique, whilst holding the needle mounted on the needle holder. The surgeon will thus be using a loop of thread, much as you would when sewing clothing. This technique requires a certain amount of practice. Before the operation begins, you should ask the local staff to show you how this is done, since when the needle requires rethreading, you may need to do it for the surgeon. The only available suture materials may be silk, nylon and catgut, and the needles, may be blunt, so excessive force may be required in their use. This both traumatises the tissues and makes the operation hazardous.

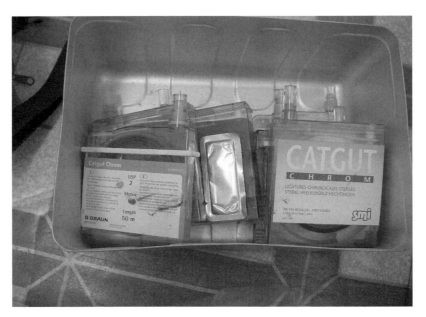

**Figure 21.1** Sutures in the developing world. Note that the suture materials are stored on spools. They require threading onto a needle.

## Instrument, swab and pack counts

Counting these surgical materials to ensure none is left in the patient, is an essential part of any developed world operation. However, in the developing world there may not be instrument counts and even if done, they may not be accurate. To make matters more critical, most of the packs and swabs used in the developing world do not have radio-opaque thread within them, so cannot be detected on post-operative X-ray.

Therefore it is essential that the surgeon and you, the assistant keep a constant mental note of the whereabouts of swabs, particularly abdominal packs during intra-abdominal operations.

## The patient

Consent and patient identification need to be checked. The western system of consent may need modification for local conditions. Generally this is managed by the local authorities. It should be remembered that many people are illiterate. It is best to agree upon and mark the operative site with the patient and relatives pre-operatively.

In many cultures, patients themselves may not necessarily make the decision as to whether they can undergo operation. The decision-maker may be a family elder. The operation may need to be postponed, to await the arrival of the necessary person. This becomes difficult when the patient needs an urgent procedure. Advice should be sought from the local staff, but generally an *operation should not proceed* if there is any doubt on the matter, and particularly if no one will take responsibility for the decision to proceed. If this principle is not observed, you may find yourself in the same category as the surgeon (local people will not differentiate these positions), and be regarded as having proceeded without consent. Even if the patient's life is saved, this may potentially be viewed as a grave disregard for local authority.

## The operation

Surgical staff from the developed world are often amazed at what surgery can be done, and what excellent results can be achieved in the developing world, often under very difficult circumstances. It is a tribute to those who work there.

The pathology which presents to surgical teams in the developing world is generally gross and the surgery life-changing. It is likely that you will see conditions that you have previously never seen in the developed world, or if so, not in such a florid form. You need to be versatile, resourceful and innovative in your

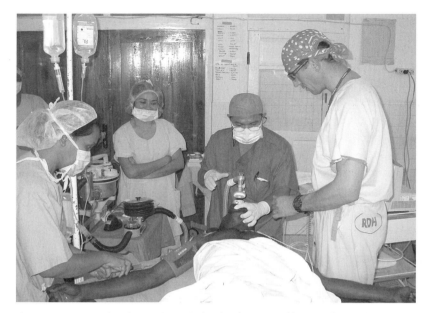

**Figure 21.2** Operating theatre scene in the developing world. General anaesthesia using ether. This is being administered via an EMO vaporizer (a simple, robust and reliable machine), and associated hand bellows. The hand-written word lists on the wall in the background were used as an aide memoir between languages.

approach. Treatment may require modification of equipment, 'lateral thinking' and appropriate application of surgical principles (see Figure 21.2).

Often there is no qualified anaesthetist, with anaesthesia being supplied by nursing staff or the surgeon.

Ketamine is a safe and commonly used agent. You need to be aware of the peculiarities of this form of anaesthesia. Patients commonly have their eyes open, and may vocalise (sometimes loudly), and have grimacing and arm and leg movements. One soon becomes familiar with these and learns to operate accordingly. These effects are outweighed by the safety, cost effectiveness and versatility of ketamine in this setting. Other anaesthetic agents with which you may not be familiar, such as ether and halothane, may also be used in the developing world.

## The local surgical staff

Perhaps the best aspect of surgical work in the developing world is meeting and working with the local surgical theatre staff. Most are wonderful people, operating under less than ideal circumstances, who are willing to teach you, and similarly to learn from your presence. They will probably teach you patience, instil a sense of realism, and show what can be achieved with minimal investigations and good clinical and surgical skills, at minimal cost. You may question the expenditure on the western health system thereafter.

## ■ Recommendations before a visit to the developing world

1 Speak at length with those who have worked in such situations.
2 Ascertain whether you think this type of work is for you, and whether you can cope. If you think you cannot, it is better not to start, and acknowledge that this is not for you. If you are unsure, select *a short visit* to the developing world and accept that you will stick it out whatever happens.
3 Undertake assisting in a wide range of surgery *before* travelling to the developing world.
4 Undergo a full range of personal immunisations and disease prophylaxis.
5 Read as much as possible on the subject, including:
King M, Bewes P, Cairns J, and Thornton J (eds). *Primary Surgery* (Vols 1 and 2). Oxford University Press.
Or online free: www.meb.uni-bonn.de/dtc/primsurg
(Special reference to Preface by Maurice King.)
Various authors. *Surgical care at the district hospital.* World Health Organisation, 2003.
ISBN 92 4 154575 5 http://bookorders.who.int/bookorders/anglais

## Summary

Surgical work in the developing world is likely to be some of the most rewarding and memorable in your career and requires resourcefulness, innovation and tolerance. It is an opportunity to meet and work with some great people in situations which they regard as normal; but to you, at least initially, are 'outside your comfort zone'.

## 22

# Vascular surgery: (1) Open surgery

**Phil Puckridge** MBBS FRACS

Waikato District Hospital, Hamilton, New Zealand

Familiarity and experience often makes the best assistants, but like most things you cannot become experienced without assisting first! There are general principles for any assistant when first assisting, which apply equally to vascular surgery. These include making yourself familiar with the anatomy of the area being operated on, reviewing the surgical procedure being performed, and becoming familiar with the different instruments that will be encountered in vascular surgery. Finally, it is useful to ask about the surgeon and his preferences prior to the operation.

As a surgical assistant it is usually polite to meet the patient before the operation. This is especially important if he or she will receive a bill from you, or on your behalf.

## ■ General principles

### Open operations

The specialty of vascular surgery encompasses arterial and venous surgery, and some related operations such as amputations. This chapter deals mainly with arterial surgery, because it is in this type of surgery that the assistant needs special skills, which are seldom needed elsewhere. However these skills are also applicable to venous surgery.

There are several important steps that are common to most arterial operations. These are: exposure of the vessels, establishing 'control' of vessels; temporary occlusion of the vessels, and the therapeutic part of the operation, which may involve grafting, patching, or performing anastomoses. These steps, and the assistant's role in them, are described in more detail below.

### Exposure

Most vascular procedures start by exposing the vessels required for the operation to be performed. During the operation, the surgeon must be able to stop blood flowing from 'upstream or downstream' to the operative site, whenever needed.

This is known as 'control' of the vessel. Therefore, the exposure must be not only of the diseased segment being treated, but also of the vessel proximal and distal to that segment. Achieving proper exposure is often the most exacting and time-consuming part of vascular surgery.

Depending on the operation and site of surgery, exposure may vary from relatively small incisions over the carotid or femoral vessels, to laparotomy and thoraco-abdominal approaches to the aorta. It is important to be familiar with different instrument and requirements for each of these approaches.

As in many other forms of surgery, a self-retaining retractor is often placed in the wound, to retract the superficial tissues and allow vision as well as applying tension to the tissues around a vessel. These vary in size from small to large table-mounted types (see p. 75).

As an assistant, you can help the surgeon expose a vessel by using forceps to grasp the tissue next to the vessel. Retract this tissue away from the vessel. This is known as counter-traction and is an important surgical principle (see also ch. 9, p. 51). Counter-traction puts the tissue under tension and allows easier dissection of the vessel. Most commonly, the surgeon and assistant stand on opposite sides of the operating table. Therefore, most commonly, you will usually be retracting the tissue on your side of a vessel, towards yourself. The surgeon is then able to apply counter-traction on the opposite site.

Importantly, do not grasp the vessel itself unless specifically instructed; this can damage the vessel. This is a key principle of vascular surgery: the surgeon aims to dissect the body away from the vessel without manipulating the vessel itself. Sometimes this is stated as a surgical maxim: 'dissect the body off the vessels, not the vessels off the body'.

## Control of vessels

It hardly needs to be stated, that operations on large blood vessels can potentially result in the patient losing large volumes of blood quickly. Therefore, during an operation, the surgeon needs to be able to find a vessel quickly, and to stop or slow blood flow through it, even if it is covered in a pool of blood or other fluid that obscures the view. This is known as having 'control' of the vessel.

Regardless of the vessel involved, obtaining control of vessels is usually performed proximally and distally, by passing silastic or rubber slings around them. These slings are often called 'vessel loops'. Once a loop is slung around a vessel, the surgeon can stop or slow the flow of blood through it whenever required. This is done by simply pulling upwards on the loop, thereby kinking the vessel.

After dissecting the vessel free from the surrounding tissue, the surgeon will pass a right-angled clamp or grasper (e.g. a Mixter) under it. The assistant should pass the vessel loop to the grasper end first using forceps (see also Figure 10.24, and 'loaded ties', pp. 85–6). This ensures that as the vessel loop is pulled underneath the vessel, the likelihood of it catching on tissue is reduced. After it has been placed, a loop is usually secured by clipping its two free ends together with an artery clip.

## Temporary occlusion of vessels

After control of the vessels has been obtained, the vessel being operated on is temporary occluded. This allows the vessel to be opened without bleeding, which in turn allows good surgical access to the interior of the artery. Temporary occlusion is done by a variety of methods as outlined below.

### Clamping

Arterial clamps can be applied to the vessel in either a vertical or horizontal direction, depending on the circumstances. These clamps are designed to be gentle on the vessels; the ratchet should be closed only enough to stop the flow of blood. Forcible closure beyond this is unnecessary and may damage the artery, especially if it is heavily calcified. A useful technique to understand the force of arterial clamps, is to close one of them on your own web space between the thumb and index finger. This is not painful, and demonstrates well the gentleness of this type of instrument. An arterial clamp is a specialised instrument, which should not be confused with a standard 'artery clip' (haemostat). The standard artery clip is designed to crush tissue, and would cause considerable pain, were you to close it on your web space.

Because the range of arterial operations is wide, it is unsurprising that arterial clamps are available in many different shapes and sizes, and suited to different purposes. They range in size from small 'bulldog' clips, about the same size as a paper-clip, to large clamps for the aorta.

### Occlusion balloons

These are often useful in very calcified arteries, where clamping may result in fracture of atherosclerotic plaques and damage to the artery. The catheter is passed into the artery and the balloon inflated to obstruct the flow of blood.

There are various balloons manufactured specifically for this purpose. Alternatively, some surgeons simply use a Fogarty catheter with a tap applied to the end. The tap allows the balloon to be inflated with an appropriate volume of saline, after which the tap is closed to keep the balloon inflated.

### Tourniquet exsanguination technique

The vessels of the calf and foot are delicate, and sometimes damaged by clamping. The tourniquet exsanguination technique allows those vessels to be opened without the need for clamping. There are several variations, but the following is the method the author uses on the lower leg during distal bypass surgery. The technique can be adapted for use on an upper limb.

After elevating the leg, a type of rubber bandage, known as an Esmarch bandage, is wound around the leg from the foot upwards. This exsanguinates the leg by pushing blood out of the venous system. When the thigh is reached, a gauze pack is placed around the thigh to protect the skin, and the Esmarch bandage is tightly wound around multiple times, to form an arterial tourniquet.

### Flow occluders

These instruments are placed within the artery to occlude flow. They are designed for use in small vessels. Some have a central channel to allow flow through the occluder.

## The 'therapeutic' part of the operation.

### Grafts

These may be of artificial material ('prosthetic graft'), or may be fashioned from one of the patient's own veins ('autologous vein graft').

*Prosthetic grafts*

These are manufactured in a wide variety of different materials, and it is beyond the capacity of this text to describe these in detail. Like any artificial material introduced into the body, a prosthetic graft is a foreign body, albeit a therapeutic one. Therefore, it should be handled as little as possible to avoid contamination. (see also prothetic materials, p. 90).

*Autologous vein grafts*

The great saphenous vein is the usual conduit of choice for vein bypass. However, other veins can also be used, such as the short saphenous, and arm veins, such as the cephalic and basilic. Harvesting of vein follows the same principles as exposure of any vessel, as described above. It can be performed either by making an incision along the length of the vein, or by 'skip incisions', which leave skin bridges between a series of incisions. There are also new endoscopic techniques. If skip incisions are used, a Langenbeck retractor is inserted under the skin bridge, to allow the surgeon better access to the vein. A wide Langenbeck retractor is better suited to this purpose.

When a vein is harvested for use as an arterial conduit, it will almost always have multiple small tributaries, which must be ligated. As the harvest proceeds, most vascular surgeons ligate the tributaries 'in continuity', which means that before the tributary is divided, it is ligated proximally and distally. A common ligature is 3-0 polyglactic acid ('Vicryl'). The surgeon passes a right-angled forceps (e.g. 'Mixter forceps', see Figure 10.11, p. 66) under the tributary and the assistant passes a tie (ligature) to it using forceps. The tip of the tie should be placed in the surgeon's open forceps, for the surgeon to grasp and pull through.

The side next to the vein being harvested is tied first, and the 'body side' second. Rather than simply cutting both ends of the tie short, most surgeons will ask that you cut one of them longer (about 10 or 15 cm); this allows you to use the tie itself as a retractor.

By gently retracting on the tie, you draw the tributary away from the tissues, so providing more space for the surgeon to apply the next tie. To save time, some surgeons will use a small metal clip, such as a 'ligaclip', instead of the second tie. After the second ligature (or a clip) is placed on the 'body side' of the tributary, the surgeon cuts the tributary between the ligatures. You may then cut the remaining suture material as appropriate; normally the surgeon will not do this, because the scissors used for cutting the vein may be damaged by cutting suture material (see pp. 55–9).

### Handling veins

The intima of veins (their internal lining) is so delicate, that even the gentlest grasping of a vein with forceps will damage it. Therefore, if you are required to retract a vein (e.g. to apply counter-traction, while the surgeon dissects the vein out from its surrounding tissues), how are you to do so? The solution is to use forceps to grasp the fascia adjacent to the vein, rather than the vein itself. Alternatively, retract the vein with a vessel loop passed around it, or with your fingers.

After the vein is harvested, it is temporarily stored in heparinised saline, either in a wet swab or in a bowl. The heparinised saline should either be warm (body temperature), or room temperature.

### Checking for leaks prior to insertion

Most tributaries are ligated as soon as they are encountered, while the vein is being harvested from the leg (or arm). However, some tributaries will only be noticeable when the vein is checked for leaks, prior to inserting it into the patient. The surgeon checks for leaks by gently distending the vein with heparinised saline. Larger tributaries detected in this way may be grasped by a mosquito clamp and gently held by the assistant, allowing the surgeon to ligate the tributary. Smaller leaks require suturing. While the surgeon does this, it is helpful for you, the assistant, to hold the vein still. Gently press on the vein with your fingers, fixing it in place against the operating surface.

### Placement of graft in the patient

Several different methods are used. The two basic methods are:

1 The reversed vein graft. The vein is removed from its original location, and placed in the desired new site. The term 'reversed' is used, because veins contain one-way valves. Therefore, simply reversing the vein's direction allows blood to flow through it, without needing to destroy the valves.

2 The *in-situ* vein graft or non-reversed graft. In the *in-situ* method, the vein is not removed from its original location. A non-reversed graft is moved from its original position, but not reversed from its original orientation. Obviously, for blood flow to occur in *in-situ* or non-reversed vein grafts, the valves must be destroyed. This is done using instruments called valvulotomes. There are several different types of these instruments, but from the assistant's viewpoint, they are all similar. They are all threaded up the vein, and then cut the valves when withdrawn. To check that the valves have successfully been destroyed, the surgeon may either use a fibre-optic angioscope to look at the valves directly, or perform an angiogram or ultrasound prior to completing the operation.

Whichever technique is used, it is important for the assistant to help and ensure that the vein graft is not twisted when placed in the patient.

## Suturing vessels: anastomoses and vessel patches

Obviously, after an artery has been opened during the course of an operation, it must be closed again. This is usually done either by joining it to another artery or graft (i.e. an anastomosis), or by suturing in a patch of some other material (usually vein). In both of these situations, the vascular surgeon will usually use a monofilament suture, such as polypropylene ('Prolene'). Depending on the size of the vessel, the suture will vary in size from 3/0 for aortic surgery to 7/0 or 8/0 for small vessels. A double-ended suture (i.e. needle at each end of the suture) is used.

Vascular anastomoses are mostly performed using a continuous suture technique. (However, in paediatric patients and some micro-vascular situations, interrupted sutures are used.) Whether the surgeon is performing an anastomosis or a patch, from the assistant's viewpoint, the technique is quite similar.

A common method is for the surgeon to place a suture through the apex of the graft (or patch), and through a corresponding point of the arteriotomy. Because there is a needle on each end of the suture, the surgeon can then run two continuous suture lines away from the apex; first along one side, then the other.

A second common method of performing anastomoses is the 'parachute' technique. In this technique, the graft (or patch) and target vessel are held a few centimetres apart, while the surgeon places the sutures in them; this allows the sutures to be placed accurately under direct vision. The graft or patch is then 'parachuted' down to the artery and the anastomosis completed (see also 'handling multiple clipped sutures', p. 61 and Figure 10.7, p. 62).

### The assistant's role

Because the suture material used in vascular surgery is often fine diameter, it is particularly prone to break if mis-handled, for example by snagging on clamps surrounding the operative field. It is therefore particularly important that you help prevent breakage. Do this firstly by covering potential snagging points with moistened towels, ensuring a balance between covering the instruments and obscuring the surgical field. Secondly, hold the suture material out of the surgeon's way, using the technique known as 'following' the suture (see p. 88).

If the surgeon is using the parachute technique (see above), it is important that initially when 'following', you simply hold the suture loosely out of the way, applying little or no tension to it. Applying tension will tend to pull the graft and artery together before the surgeon desires it. Only after the surgeon has snugged the anastomosis down, should you apply tension when following the suture.

The same principles of 'following' a suture in any other situation, also apply in vascular surgery. For example, the surgeon will often place the suture in your hand at the tension he or she desires, and in the position that is most favourable. Also, it is important not to reach across the surgeon's field of vision to grasp the suture.

Generally, when 'following' a suture, you should hold the suture away on the same side of the anastomosis that the surgeon is working on. That is, do not allow the suture material to pass across the anastomosis. As suturing goes around the 'heel' or 'toe' of the anastomosis, change hands to avoid reaching across the operating field.

Apply constant, even tension so that there is no slacking of the suture line, which can cause leaking of the anastomosis after completion. Some surgeons say you should be able to 'play' the suture as if it were a guitar string. However, if you apply too much tension, you risk ripping the suture out of the arterial wall, or breaking the suture, both of which you will quickly feel unhappy about.

The smaller the vessel, the more delicate it is, and the finer (and more breakable) the suture material that is used. Therefore, for smaller vessels, less tension is needed, and communication between assistant and surgeon regarding the appropriate amount of tension becomes even more important.

When the surgeon has almost finished the anastomosis, he or she will usually clear clot and debris from the vessels by 'back-bleeding' them and flushing them with heparinised saline. The surgeon will then insert the final few sutures to close the anastomosis. At this point, if you hold both sutures up away from the suture line, as if 'following', you can help the edges of the graft and vessel sit in such a way as to make the final sutures easier for the surgeon.

### Squirting the surgeon's hands

During an operation, dried blood accumulates on the surgeon's gloves and on the suture material. This makes the suture sticky and liable to catch when tying knots. If this occurs, a small suture, such as 6/0 will often break, leading to the assistant once again feeling unhappy. This is avoided by wetting the gloves and suture material.

As the assistant, you may be required to provide this wetting effect, by squirting saline onto the surgeon's hands as the knot is being tied, and just before. This is done with a syringe, which the scrub nurse will give you. Some people seem to feel uncomfortable with the idea of squirting water onto their senior colleagues, and only squirt it onto the suture material itself. This should be avoided. Consciously aim to squirt water onto the fingers of the surgeon's knot-tying hand, and the hand itself.

# ■ Specific situations in vascular surgery

## Carotid surgery

During carotid surgery it is vitally important that you do not handle the tissues roughly, especially the carotid artery itself. Rough handling of the carotid artery can lead to dislodgement of atherosclerotic emboli that could result in a stroke.

A useful assisting technique in carotid surgery, is to use a fine sucker to clear blood, instead of mopping it up with gauze packs or swabs. This allows delicacy and provides a blood-free field for the surgeon. When doing this in the arterial lumen, it is very important to avoid touching the luminal surface with the tip of the sucker. If the inner surface of the artery is caught in the sucker it can be damaged.

If blood has clotted over the field obscuring the view, wash with heparinised saline and suction the fluid away. Once again, this avoids inadvertent movement of the carotid artery.

During carotid endarterectomy (an operation where the diseased lining of the artery is removed), while the artery is opened, irrigate its surface regularly to wash any accumulating fibrin or blood clot from the surface. This prevents formation of adherent clot which might embolise when the circulation is restored.

## Aortic surgery

At the beginning of the case and during initial dissection of the retroperitoneum, if you retract the mesocolon with a medium-sized Deaver retractor, you will greatly improve exposure for the surgeon. It is especially important to do this well during repair of a ruptured aortic aneurysm, as it allows exposure and helps keep the bowel out of the way. Obviously, the aorta and its terminating vessels (the common iliacs) are big vessels, so the sutures used for anastomoses are also relatively big. Therefore, when 'following' a suture during the anastomoses, slightly greater tension is allowed and will help keep the anastomosis blood-tight.

# 23 Vascular surgery: (2) Endovascular surgery

**Kath Phillips** RGON

Specialist Radiology Nurse, Waikato District Hospital, Hamilton, New Zealand

**Phil Puckridge** MBBS FRACS

Consultant Vascular Surgeon, Waikato District Hospital, Hamilton, New Zealand

Endovascular surgery is an exciting field in which rapid advances are currently being made. It is very different to open vascular surgery, and a different set of assisting skills and techniques is required. Highly specialised equipment is also necessary, so procedures usually take place either in an angiography suite (sometimes known as a 'cath-lab'), or in a custom-built endovascular theatre. It is essential to work in these areas to gain the required skills. For all these reasons, it is beyond the scope of this chapter to provide a definitive guide on how to assist at all such procedures. Instead, it is intended to give the reader an overview of endovascular procedures and how they are performed, together with some of the general principles of assisting at these procedures.

## ■ Introduction

Procedures may be broadly categorised into purely diagnostic studies (angiography) and therapeutic ('interventional') procedures. Most procedures take place under local anaesthetic.

A variety of specialists perform endovascular procedures including vascular surgeons, interventional radiologists and cardiologists. Often for complex procedures, two specialists may work together.

Because X-ray radiation is used during the procedures, knowledge about radiation safety is essential. A lead gown and a cumulative-radiation exposure tag are required when present at these procedures. It is important to remember that the further from the source of the X-ray beam, the less radiation exposure received. This is due to the 'inverse square rule', which means, for example, by being positioned 2 m from the radiation source, instead of 1 m, the radiation exposure is quartered.

Although endovascular procedures are considered less invasive than open surgery, there is still considerable potential for patient injury. Injuries can occur due to damage to the vessel wall resulting in thromboembolic events, vessel wall dissections, and intravascular migration of equipment, or contrast reactions (see below).

## ■ Medical preparation of the patient

Patients with impaired renal or cardiac function need careful fluid management to avoid fluid overload. Iodinated contrast agents can worsen renal function and in this situation metformin (a medication used for diabetics) can lead to serious adverse reactions. Consequently, metformin is usually stopped 24–48 h before the procedure. Patients are pre-hydrated as preparation for the procedure if renal function is abnormal. Poorly controlled hypertension increases the risk of post-procedure bleeding. Anticoagulants increase the risk of bleeding so are usually withheld.

Patients should be able to lie flat for a minimum of 2 h post-procedure, to allow the puncture site to clot effectively. Longer rest times of up to 4 h are needed after interventional procedures, such as angioplasty and stenting. However, newer percutaneous closure devices allow immediate mobilisation.

Allergy to contrast or to other iodine-containing substances does not necessarily contraindicate the procedure, but some patients may need pre-medication with steroids and antihistamines.

## ■ Endovascular access

Most endovascular procedures begin by using the Seldinger technique to access the vessel. In this technique, a needle puncture is made in a peripheral artery. This will usually be the femoral artery, but other arteries such as the radial or brachial may be used. A guide wire is then fed through the needle puncture into the arterial lumen, and a catheter is passed over the wire.

## ■ Endovascular procedures

The wire and catheter are manipulated into the appropriate position to inject contrast media and acquire images of the vessels. The next steps depend on the type of procedure being undertaken and include procedures to enlarge narrow arteries by angioplasty or stenting; embolisation procedures to occlude unwanted vessels such as aneurysmal vessels or those supplying tumours; and procedures to repair abdominal aortic aneurysms.

Local anaesthetic is used to anaesthetise the puncture site. Most patients find these procedures painless once this has taken effect and access has been gained. Sudden discomfort or pain is a warning that something is amiss, and the operator will usually take steps to investigate further.

## ■ Handling catheters and wires

There is a very large variety of catheters and wires, and it is beyond the scope of this text to describe them all. You should aim to familiarise yourself with the types used in 'your' cath-lab. Briefly, catheters and wires vary widely in their size, shape, stiffness, and coating based on the purpose for which they are designed. Catheters also vary in the number, size and location of holes at their tips. As with most other single-use medical devices, their packaging usually contains helpful and detailed information about the product.

There are two principal methods of inserting catheters and balloons along the wires due to design differences in catheters and wire technology:

1 In the 'over the wire' technique, the catheter is fed along the wire *through its central lumen*. The wire should project from the end of the catheter, before the catheter enters the patient. Otherwise it is possible to push the wire in with the catheter, and inadvertently lose the wire inside the patient. It is an important job of the assistant to ensure this doesn't happen.

2 In the 'rapid exchange' or 'monorail' method, the wire is fed into the end of the catheter, and exits a side-port midway down the catheter, which then runs along rather like a monorail train. When you are assisting at this method, it is important to keep the wire straight, to ensure a smooth run along the wire. The wires are very fine in monorail systems (usually 0.014–0.018 in. diameter), and easily kinked, but this must be avoided because the catheter will then not slide properly.

Many of these wires are very springy. Therefore, you should handle them carefully and keep them coiled in a smooth, large-diameter coil (e.g. 20–30 cm). Otherwise, the wires can suddenly flick or drop off the sterile area and become contaminated. Also, you should aim to keep the wire fixed in position when the operator is trying to catheterise a target vessel, and when exchanging catheters. Do this by pinning it against a sterile surface with your fingers.

# ■ Preparing equipment

As with any other medical procedure, anticipation (see p. 25) is important. In this setting, anticipation means that any equipment that is likely to be needed should be readily available. Also, you should be familiar with the steps of a procedure, so that as it proceeds, you can predict which step will come next and prepare for it. This is especially important when working on cerebral vessels, where it is essential that minimal time is taken, to avoid possible brain ischaemia.

Catheters or dilators with a lumen should be pre-flushed with heparinised saline. Ensure there is no debris or air bubbles in the lumen, as even small micro-emboli can have devastating effects in an arterial system.

During the procedures, intermittent flushing of all equipment and sheaths is essential to avoid clot formation. This is generally performed using heparinised saline. The concentration of heparinised saline may vary between differing institutions, so care should be taken to be familiar with the local protocols. There are two different ways to perform the flushing of equipment and sheaths in the patient:

1 *The 'closed system'*: A special pump is primed with heparinised saline, which it then injects at set intervals to ensure there is no stasis in the catheters. This has the additional advantage of lowering the risk of possible air emboli.

2 *The 'open system'*: This usually means that the system is flushed by hand, using syringes filled with heparinised saline. If so, ensure that the syringe has no air bubbles in it. Also, always hold the syringe upright while injecting, so that if any bubbles are present, they will tend to stay in the syringe rather than be flushed through it.

# ■ Specialised equipment: balloons, stents, etc.

With most of these devices, the preparation is important, and specific to each device, so again, you should familiarise yourself with the devices being used before assisting at procedures. The medical companies that provide the equipment have clinical specialists that will assist with education and are an important resource.

When preparing catheters and balloons for insertion, always inspect the entire length of the catheter to ensure there are no kinks, cracks or debris. The lumen should be flushed with heparinised saline.

Angioplasty balloons should be prepared by applying suction to the hub to ensure all air is removed. There should be contrast in the hub, so that when the balloon is inflated it is easy to visualise. When deflating the balloon, keep a negative pressure on the balloon so that it withdraws easily and has the lowest possible profile.

There are two basic types of stent: self-expanding and balloon-mounted. Preparation of stents involves inspecting the mechanism to ensure it is intact. Do not handle the stent, as this may cause dislodgement or even accidental deployment.

Distal protection devices are increasingly being used when working in arteries supplying organs that tolerate embolism poorly (e.g. the carotid and renal arteries). Among the wide variety of designs are occlusion balloons and net or basket-like devices. They are placed distal to the target lesion to trap emboli, and are removed at the end of the procedure.

## ■ Endovascular repair of abdominal aneurysms

This method of repairing abdominal aneurysms offers the advantage over open surgery, of avoiding laparotomy. This lessens the physiological insult to the body, leading to faster recovery (typically only 2–3 days in hospital). It is especially beneficial to patients in whom an abdominal approach would be difficult (e.g. those with severe adhesions and those who otherwise would be too unwell to tolerate major abdominal surgery). At the time of writing, the endovascular repair of abdominal aortic aneurysms is a well accepted technique that in many centres is the preferred method of repair. The disadvantages are that the devices may develop leaks ('endoleaks') and consequently, patients must be followed up indefinitely with periodic radiological surveillance by ultrasound or CT. Lastly, not all aneurysms are anatomically suitable for this method.

These devices are quite large (18–26 Fr), so access to the femoral vessels is either by open surgical cut-down or a specialised percutaneous access and closure device.

## ■ Embolisation

An embolisation procedure is the deliberate occlusion of an unwanted vessel, by injecting it with something that encourages thrombosis. Indications include bleeding from pelvic vessels in complex pelvic fractures, various small aneurysms in specific locations and elective procedures for endoleaks (see above), arterio-venous malformations, or occasionally vessels supplying tumours.

Injected agents include fine metal coils covered with tiny fibres (which encourage thrombus formation), as well as substances such as gel foam, polyvinyl chloride beads, and absolute alcohol. Whichever agent is used, you must ensure the catheter has no side holes. If side holes are present, coils can stick in them, causing the catheter to recoil, and risking migration of the coil to a vessel other than the target vessel. Similarly, alcohol and other substances can spill out unless you have a catheter with a single end hole properly placed in the target vessel.

If absolute alcohol is used, warn both the patient and the staff that the patient may smell strongly of alcohol for a few hours post-procedure. There are other complications of embolising vessels that the medical staff performing the procedure will discuss with the patient prior to the procedure.

# Immediately after the operation

# Part IV

# Immediately after the operation

At the end of any operation, the author's first inclination is to bolt to the tea-room at the earliest opportunity, and eat all the muffins before someone else does. However, it is best not to do this too often because it will certainly be noticed, even if it is not commented upon.

Instead, it is better to help with some of the innumerable small jobs to be done after any operation. Put the X-rays back in their packet, ideally in their proper order. Help wheel in the patient's bed, and help transfer the patient onto it from the operating table, especially if he or she is heavy. Fill in forms, such as histopathology request forms or audit forms. In a day-surgery unit, you may write a short discharge summary or coding report.

It is possible you may prescribe the patient's drugs or non-drug treatment orders. In this setting, drugs may be classified into the patient's usual medications (e.g. antihypertensives), and additional or alternative medications he or she may need perioperatively. Regarding the patient's usual drugs, it is very important to note that some should be continued, some temporarily withheld, and others given in a modified form. As examples, typically antihypertensives are continued, anticoagulants are temporarily withheld, and oral hypoglycaemics are replaced by subcutaneous insulin. Additional drugs may include antiemetics, analgesics, antibiotics, and prophylactic anticoagulants, such as subcutaneous heparin injections. Intravenous or other fluids may also be placed in this category.

Non-drug treatment orders include observations (routine including heart rate, blood pressure, respiratory and temperature or 'special' observations such as neurovascular observations), fasting status, drain management, special requirements for positioning the patient, and coughing and breathing exercises.

If the case is anything other than a minor one, and especially if the operation is during a long inpatient stay, it is good practice to make a brief entry in large letters, in the patient's case-notes. This makes it much easier in future to make a rapid assessment of the case-notes, even for someone who is unfamiliar with the patient. It is not necessary to write all the details of the operation, provided of course that a proper operation note is made elsewhere. For example:

| 3/9/2005 22:45 | OPERATION |
|---|---|

Laparotomy, oversewing perforated duodenal ulcer
　See formal operation note.

The usual custom is for the doctor who does the operation, to write the formal operation record. However, if the surgeon you are assisting is ignoring this custom, you may be asked to write it. Writing a good description of an operative procedure takes practice, and it is unlikely that as a novice you will suddenly be asked to write the operation note for a major operation.

Different hospitals have different systems for recording operation notes. The three common methods are:

1　Hand-write the note on a special sheet provided in the operating theatre (often with carbon copies).
2　Type the note on a computer in the operating theatre, and print it out.
3　Dictate the note into a dictation device.

Use a systematic approach to writing operation records. Essentially, try to make brief notes that summarise what was done. Using point form makes it easier to read. Briefly describe the position of the patient first (e.g. supine, lithotomy position). Most surgeons then use the 'IF P.C.' method, consciously or otherwise. That is, describe the *I*ncision (e.g. upper midline in the abdomen, transverse skin crease in the neck). Next, describe the operative *F*indings. That is, describe the pathology and any significant negative findings. For example, in a resection of a colon cancer, describe the site of the cancer, whether it was mobile or attached to adjacent structures, whether there was any extra-colonic spread (especially to the liver), and which important structures were seen and protected. If there were any significant incidental findings (e.g. a Meckel's diverticulum), include this in the note.

Then describe the *P*rocedure itself. Was it an incision (e.g. of an abscess), an excision, an exploration or some other category of operation (see p. 33). A good test of your description is to imagine that another surgeon is to re-operate on the patient in future for some reason, and your note will be the only information available about the operation. Would he or she understand what was done, and why? Then describe the method and suture material used to *C*lose the wound.

Once the above tasks have been completed, and if you are really good, you might help mop the floors. Unfortunately in the operating theatre, humility is a commodity that is often in short supply, so mopping the floors will usually bring forth surprise and admiration from the other staff present. However, you should aim to be humble without being obsequious, and confident without being arrogant.

If you are contemplating a career in surgery, you may keep a logbook of the operations at which you assist. Indeed, in most surgical training schemes such a logbook is compulsory. Information can be recorded on a simple sheet of paper carried in your wallet, and transferred to a folder once filled. Alternatively, some surgeons use an electronic auditing system, entering patient and operation details in a hand-held or laptop computer. These systems offer the advantage that data can easily be manipulated. For example, logbook summaries can be generated quickly and easily. Whichever method you choose, by far the best way is to record the details while they are still fresh in your mind: either immediately after the operation or the same evening.

If the surgeon you are assisting will shortly be doing another operation to follow the one you have just finished, your time may be better spent leaving the theatre to introduce yourself to the next patient.

# Glossary

### Abdominal aortic aneurysm (AAA)
A condition in which the abdominal aorta expands in diameter from its usual size of approximately the size of its owner's thumb to several cm. The major complication is rupture, which usually causes catastrophic blood loss and very often, prompt death.

### Adhesions
Scar tissue in a hollow space (especially the abdomen), causing two surfaces that are normally separated, to adhere to one another.

### Anastomosis
A join (especially a surgical join) between two hollow structures, for example between the small bowel and the colon after the right colon has been removed (right hemicolectomy).

### Anterior superior iliac spine (ASIS)
The anterior and lateral bony prominence of the pelvis.

### Appose (verb)
To bring two structures together so they lie next to each other, in contact.

### Balanced salt solution (BSS)
A special fluid, designed to maintain corneal epithelial and endothelial integrity during intraocular surgery.

### Barium enema
An investigation to examine the colon, in which radio-opaque material (barium sulphate paste) is given as an enema, followed by abdominal X-rays.

## Betadine

A trade-name of an iodine-containing antiseptic solution.

## Chlorhexidine

An antiseptic solution.

## Cholecystectomy

An operation to remove the gallbladder. It is most commonly performed laparoscopically.

## Colonoscopy

An examination of the colon. A long flexible tube with a television camera attached is inserted into the anus and manipulated through the colon.

## Consultant

A fully trained specialist doctor, appointed to a hospital (especially a training hospital). The consultant usually bears ultimate responsibility for decisions about the patient's care.

## Continuous suture (*cf.* interrupted suture, below)

A common method of suturing whereby a single length of suture is sewn back and forth between the two objects, approximately forming a spiral.

## CT scan

An abbreviation of Computerised Tomography. A special machine uses X-rays to make images of the body and internal organs, as though the body had been sliced like a loaf of bread.

## Depth of field

A photographic term used to describe how much of a picture is in focus. For example, imagine you are standing in the front row of a large concert, and taking a photograph of the crowd behind you. Using a broad depth of field, the faces of all of the people behind you would be in sharp focus. However, if you wanted to take a photograph of some friends standing five rows behind you, you might choose a narrow depth of field, so that your friends' faces were in focus, but the people behind them and in front of them were blurred.

## Distal (*cf.* proximal, below)

Further away from the point of origin (e.g. in the arm, the wrist is distal to the elbow, because it is further away from the shoulder).

### Drain (noun)

A piece of material, usually tubular plastic, inserted into the body temporarily, to drain a body fluid.

### Drain (verb)

To drain a collection of abnormal fluid (e.g. pus) from the body. This may be done via a surgical incision, or sometimes by inserting a needle.

### DVT/PE

The common abbreviation for Deep Venous Thrombosis and Pulmonary Embolus. A condition in which blood clots (DVTs) form in the deep veins (usually in the legs). The clot may break free, travelling to, and lodging in, the lungs (PE). Depending on the degree of obstruction to the flow of blood in the lungs, this may cause sudden death, chronic scarring of the lungs, or be asymptomatic.

### Enoxeparin (trade name 'Clexane')

A drug closely related to heparin (*q.v.*) but perhaps with fewer side effects.

### Eponymous

A condition or instrument named after a particular person, for example, Langenbeck's retractor, named after the German surgeon, Bernhard R.K. von Langenbeck (1810–1887).

### Extra Capsular Cataract Extraction (ECCE)

Strictly speaking, every modern cataract operation is extracapsular, because it leaves behind the crystalline lens capsule (in contrast to intracapsular cataract extractions which removed the lens capsule along with the lens). However, ECCE is used to describe procedures where the cataractous crystalline lens is removed 'en bloc'.

### Gauge (in reference to suture material)

The thickness, and therefore the strength of the suture material. In the most common gauging system, a larger numeral usually implies a thinner suture. For example, 5/0 (pronounced 'five-oh') suture material is finer than 3/0. However, anything *heavier* than 2/0 suture material is measured in single digits, but with a larger numeral implying a heavier suture. For example, suture material 1 is heavier than 0 (pronounced 'oh'). Anything heavier than 1 is seldom used.

## Heparin

A blood-thinning drug commonly given by injection at the time of surgery, for prophylaxis against DVT/PE. It has a short half-life of about 90 min. (*cf.* enoxeparin and warfarin).

## Histology

The science of examining tissues at a cellular level, using a microscope.

## Inferior (*cf.* superior, below)

Anatomical term meaning 'beneath'. For example in the face, the mouth is inferior to the nose.

## Intern (United States and Australia)

Strictly, an intern is a recent medical graduate who lives in a hospital (*cf.* an extern, who does the same job but lives off-campus). However, by convention, it is used to describe any doctor in his or her first year of practice after graduation. The term extern is now rarely used, except by pedants.

## Interrupted suture (*cf.* continuous suture, above)

A common method of suturing whereby the suture needle passes just once through each structure being sutured (or in some variations, twice) before the ends are knotted together and cut.

## Intraocular lens (IOL)

After ECCE or phaco (see entries in this glossary) has removed the diseased native lens, it is replaced with a prosthetic lens (IOL). The prosthetic lens focuses light onto the retina. It may be made of silicone, acrylic plastic, or polymethylmethacrylate (PMMA). An IOL of a total of 12 mm diameter may be delivered, folded, through a specialised injection system allowing use of a wound of 3 mm width or less.

## Irrigation and aspiration (I/A)

The infusion and removal of fluid within the eye to assist removal of cataractous material and the Ophthalmic Viscosurgical Device (OVD) from the eye.

## Ischaemia (noun)/ischaemic (adjective)

A state of inadequate blood supply, usually locally to an area of tissue and usually due to inadequate flow in the vessels supplying that tissue.

## JHO (United Kingdom)

An abbreviation for Junior House Officer. In the United Kingdom, a junior doctor equivalent to an intern (*q.v.*).

## Laparoscopy/laparoscopic surgery

The technique of inserting a specially designed viewing instrument (laparoscope) and other slim instruments into the abdominal cavity, through small incisions. The laparoscope usually has a miniature television camera attached to it, and the instruments are used to perform surgery.

## Laparotomy

Strictly speaking, this ought to mean an incision into the flank or loins (Greek 'laparo' means flank or loins). However, by convention, it instead means an incision into the peritoneal cavity, usually via the midline.

## Lateral (*cf.* medial, below)

Anatomical term meaning 'further away from the middle'. More precisely, further from the median or midsaggital plane. For example, in the face, the eye is lateral to the nose.

## Ligate/ligature

To ligate is to tie something (especially a blood vessel) so that it is no longer patent. Ligature is the piece of thread used for that purpose.

## Medial (*cf.* lateral, above)

Anatomical term meaning 'closer to the middle'. More precisely, closer to the median or midsaggital plane. For example, in the face, the nose is medial to the eye.

## Mesentery

A fatty sheet attached to some parts of the bowel, which contains its supplying blood vessels, lymphatics and nerves. The mesentery attaches the bowel to the posterior wall of the abdominal cavity.

## Mobilise

To free a structure or organ from the surrounding tissues, often in preparation for removing it.

## Necrose (verb)

In reference to a piece of living tissue, the act of it dying, or to cause it to die.

## Open procedure/open operation

The word 'open' used before the name of an operation can have subtly different meanings, depending on the context in which it is used. In abdominal operations, such as appendicectomy, it means a non-laparoscopic operation. In orthopaedic surgery, it refers to the method used to fix a fracture, where simple manipulation of the limb without incision ('closed reduction'), is not sufficient. In this context, it is often used before the words 'reduction and internal fixation', and abbreviated to ORIF. This means that the skin is incised, and the fracture is reduced and secured in an anatomical position.

## Pathologist

A medical specialist who examines tissue specimens in order to help diagnose a disease.

## Peribulbar anaesthesia

Injection of anaesthetic into the orbit to achieve ocular anaesthesia and akinesia.

## Peritoneum/peritoneal cavity

The peritoneal *cavity* is the space within the abdomen in which the intestines and other organs lie. More accurately, it is a potential space, because there is normally no 'empty space' at all, other than a few millilitres of fluid. The *peritoneum* is the lining of the peritoneal cavity. It is only a few cell-layers thick, and when healthy is smooth and glossy.

## Phacoemulsification ('phaco')

In this process, an ultrasound probe is used to emulsify the crystalline lens into a fine powder that can be removed along with fluid run through the anterior and posterior chambers of the eye. The chief advantage of this over other methods of lens extraction, is that a smaller incision can be used. This is because the incision does not need to be wide enough to allow exit of the cataractous crystalline lens 'en bloc'. The incision can therefore be so small that it does not require sutures.

## Prophylactic

A drug or other therapy given to a patient who does not have a disease, to prevent the disease from occurring (or at least decrease the chance of it). For example, prophylactic antibiotics are often given immediately before an operation, to prevent infection.

### Proximal (*cf.* distal, above)

Closer to the point of origin (e.g. in the arm, the elbow is proximal to the wrist, because it is closer to the shoulder).

### Ratchet

In surgery, the clicking mechanism on the handle of a surgical instrument, which locks the instrument's jaws in position.

### Registrar (United Kingdom and Australia)

A trainee doctor more senior than a resident (RMO/SHO), but not yet a consultant (*q.v.*). Their range of experience varies widely; some have completed all specialist training (in which case they are usually called 'senior registrar') while others have only just started it.

### Resident

This term has slightly different meanings in different countries. In Australia, it is a contraction of the term 'Resident Medical Officer' (see below); a junior doctor who is more than one year post-graduation, but not yet a registrar. It is approximately equivalent to the term Senior House Officer, which is used in the United Kingdom. In the United States, 'resident' means any trainee doctor.

### RMO

An abbreviation for Resident Medical Officer (see above, 'resident').

### Scrubbed

A person who is either taking part in a sterile operative procedure, or is immediately ready to do so, is said to be scrubbed. That is, the hands have been washed in a special way and sterile surgical gloves and a gown have been donned.

### Scrubs

The special clothing worn inside the operating theatre suite.

### SHO

An abbreviation for Senior House Officer (see above, 'resident').

### Sigmoidoscopy

An examination of the lower colon. There are two types: (a) flexible sigmoidoscopy, (which is essentially a limited version of a colonoscopy (*q.v.*)), and (b) rigid sigmoidoscopy. This uses a simple illuminated rigid tube with a small window on one end, through which the surgeon looks directly into the bowel. In this latter type, the term sigmoidoscopy is usually a misnomer, because the instrument is seldom able to reach beyond the rectum.

## Superior (*cf.* inferior, above)

Anatomical term meaning 'above'. For example in the face, the nose is superior to the mouth.

## Suture/stitch

The meanings of these two terms overlap. A 'stitch' may mean the piece of surgical thread inserted in the tissue, before, during or after the act of putting it in place. It may also refer to the act of placing the piece of thread.

'Suture' means the same thing, but may also be used to describe a length of surgical thread used for ligature.

## Torticollis

A disease affecting the sternocleidomastoid neck muscle, contracting it so that the sufferer's head is permanently or spasmodically tilted to one side.

## Trabeculectomy

An operation for glaucoma in which a controlled leak of fluid from the eye is created. The surgeon creates a partial thickness flap in the sclera, and removes a short section of the anterior chamber angle structures below it. This causes a slow leak of fluid from the eye, lowering intraocular pressure. The rate of leakage is controlled partly by the thickness of the flap. The conjunctiva is sutured back over the flap, to prevent micro-organisms from entering it.

## Trochar

A sharp spear-like instrument, which fits snugly inside a tubular surgical instrument, with its point projecting from the end. In this way, when the instrument is pushed into the tissues, the trochar cuts a hole through them. The trochar is usually then removed from the instrument. In laparoscopic surgery, trochars are used to insert ports.

## Viscoelastic or ophthalmic viscoelastic device

A viscoelastic substance, is a substance that is fluid when under pressure, but that assumes semisolid properties in the absence of pressure. Such a substance is used within the anterior and posterior chambers of the eye, to separate and maintain volume between tissue planes, such as cornea and iris, to protect delicate cells on the posterior cornea, and to lubricate the insertion of the IOL.

## Warfarin

A blood-thinning drug taken by mouth. Because it has a slow onset and offset of action (usually about three days), it is almost always temporarily withheld before all but the smallest operations(*cf.* heparin and enoxeparin).

# Suggested further reading

## ■ General principles of surgery

Chassin JL. Operative Strategy in General Surgery. Springer-Verlag, New York, 1980. Especially, Appendix A: Some Mechanical Basics of Operative Technique (p 483–496) and Appendix B: Dissecting and Sewing (p. 497–514).

Kirk RM. *Basic Surgical Techniques* (4th edition). Churchill Livingstone, Edinburgh, 1994.

## ■ Anatomy

Hollinshead WH. *Anatomy for Surgeons*, Vol 1–3. Cassell and Co Ltd, New York, 1956.

Jamieson GG. *The Anatomy of General Surgical Operations*. Churchill Livingstone, Edinburgh, 1992.

McMinn RMH. *Last's Anatomy (9th ed)*. Churchill Livingstone, Edinburgh, 1994.

## ■ Textbooks of operative surgery

Kirk RM. *General Surgical Operations* (4th edition). Churchill Livingstone, London, 2000.

McGregor IA. *Fundamental Techniques of Plastic Surgery* (8th edition). Churchill Livingstone, Edinburgh, 1989.

McLatchie GR and Leaper DJ (eds). *Oxford Handbook of Operative Surgery*. Oxford University Press, Oxford, 1996.

## ■ Miscellaneous

Anderton JM, Keen RI and Neave R. *Positioning the Surgical Patient*. Butterworths, London, 1988.

Marshall VC and Ludbrook J (eds). *Clinical Science for Surgeons* (2nd edition). Butterworths, London, 1988.

Servant C and Purkiss S. *Positioning Patients for Surgery*. Greenwich Medical Media, London, 2002.

World Health Organisation: Universal Precautions Website: http://www.who.int/hiv/topics/precautions/universal/en/

# References

Alexander JW, Fischer JE, Boyajian M, Palmquist J and Morris MJ. The influence of hair-removal methods on wound infections. *Arch. Surg.* 1983; 118: 347–352.

Arrowsmith VA, Maunder JA, Sargent RJ and Taylor R. Removal of nail polish and finger rings to prevent surgical infection. *Cochrane Database Syst. Rev.* 2001; (1): CD003325.

Bruun C. The water supply of ancient Rome. *Finn. Soc. Sci. Lett. Helsinki* 1991; 112–113.

Bulfinch T. *The Golden Age of Myth and Legend (being a revised and enlarged edition of "The Age of Fable")*. Chapter 5: Phaëton. George G. Harrap and Co. Ltd., London, 1919, pp. 51, 469.

Centres for Disease Control and Prevention. Guideline for Hand Hygiene in Health-Care Settings: Recommendations of the Healthcare Infection Control Practices Advisory Committee and HICPAC/SHEA/APIC/IDSA Hand Hygiene Task Force. MMWR 2002; 51 (no. RR-16)

Grabsch EA, Mitchell D, Hooper J and Turnidge JD. In-use efficacy of a chlorhexidine in alcohol surgical rub: a comparative study. *ANZ J. Surg.* 2004; 74: 769–772.

Lipp A and Edwards P. Disposable surgical face masks for preventing surgical wound infection in clean surgery. *Cochrane Database Syst. Rev.* 2002; (1): CD002929.

Loudon I. Why are (male) surgeons still addressed as Mr? *Brit. Med. J.* 2000; 321: 1589–1591.

Sebel PS, Bowdle TA, Ghoneim MM, Rampil IJ, Padilla RE, Gan TJ and Domino KB. The incidence of awareness during anesthesia: a multicenter United States study. *Anesth. Analg.* 2004; 99 (3): 833–839.

Tanner J and Parkinson H. Double gloving to reduce surgical cross-infection. *Cochrane Database Syst. Rev.* 2002; (3): CD003087.

# Index